# The Creative Alchemy Cycle

## ACTIVATE YOUR CREATIVITY TO WAKE UP AND GET FREE

### SARAH GREENMAN

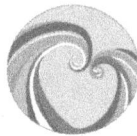

TEHOM
CENTER

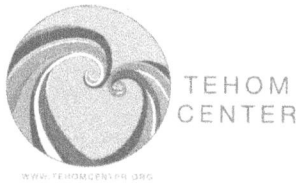

TEHOM
CENTER

*The Creative Alchemy Cycle*

Tehom Center Publishing is a 501(c)3 nonprofit publishing feminist and queer authors, with a commitment to elevate BIPOC writers. Its face and voice is Rev. Dr. Angela Yarber.

Paperback ISBN: 979-8-9914844-4-2

Ebook ISBN: 979-8-9914844-5-9

# CONTENTS

# PRAISE FOR THE CREATIVE ALCHEMY CYCLE

"Poetic, practical, and deeply relevant for these times, Sarah reminds us that our inherent creativity has the power to illuminate a more just and thriving world where the natural rhythms of Earth show us exactly how it's done."

— FLORA BOWLEY, AUTHOR OF *THE ART OF ALIVENESS*
AND *BRAVE INTUITIVE PAINTING*

"The Creative Alchemy Cycle is an essential and luminous book. Every page reveals some new delight, expanding the reader's capacities for creativity, empathy, accountability, and joy. I found myself wishing for more hours in the day to read this book: once I picked it up, it was impossible to put down. As Greenman takes readers on this surprising journey, they feel guided by the wisdom of someone who's spent a lifetime paying close attention to everything that deepens our connection to each other and ourselves. All of this is animated by nature's presence: the mystery and wonders of Earth surge from her prose."

— DR. JENNIFER ATKINSON, AUTHOR OF *GARDENLAND*
AND *THE EXISTENTIAL TOOLKIT FOR CLIMATE JUSTICE
EDUCATORS*

"In a world where our daily lives seem so fast tracked to result, performance and achievement, the beauty of this book is the invitation to slow down and turn inwards. Accompanied by Sarah's gorgeous paintings and poetry, this book is a generous nurturing gift to yourself and your creative life."

— MICKEY SUMNER, ACTOR *FRANCES HA* AND
*SNOWPIERCER*

"Though we live in different parts of Oregon, stunningly different eco systems helping us make sense of our worlds, Sarah's book offers a dynamic through line, from her place to mine (and yours). With creative supports and prompts connected to the Celtic seasonal calendar, The Creative Alchemy Cycle feels like deep rooted knowing and expansive newness all at once. Whether you, like me, are new to the Celtic seasonal cycle or a seasoned practitioner of its magic, Sarah's book will hold and inspire. In times as unbalanced and unjust as these, creative practices that connect us to the collective feel both necessary and nourishing, and this book will take you there."

— ERIN FAIRCHILD, ARTIST, ACTIVIST, AND FOUNDER
OF *JOURNAL AS ALTAR*

"Sarah Greenman's 'The Creative Alchemy Cycle' is a transformative journey that awakens the artist, changemaker, and conscientious human within us all. This powerful book stands shoulder to shoulder with works like 'Big Magic,' reinforcing the universal nature of creativity as both a practice and a way of life. Greenman's words inspire us to heighten our awareness, listen deeply, and take meaningful action. Whether you're seeking to reignite your creative spark, live in greater harmony with our planet, or enhance your relationships with others, this book serves as an indispensable source of inspiration and motivation. 'The Creative Alchemy Cycle' is more than just a read; it's a catalyst for personal growth and a beacon for those navigating their creative path. It's a must-have for anyone looking to infuse their life with purpose, creativity, and positive change."

— JACKIE LEISHMAN, ARTIST

*For my mother, whose love, creativity,
and companionship fill my life with joy.*

*And for my daughter, whose very life
is a glorious act of creative alchemy.*

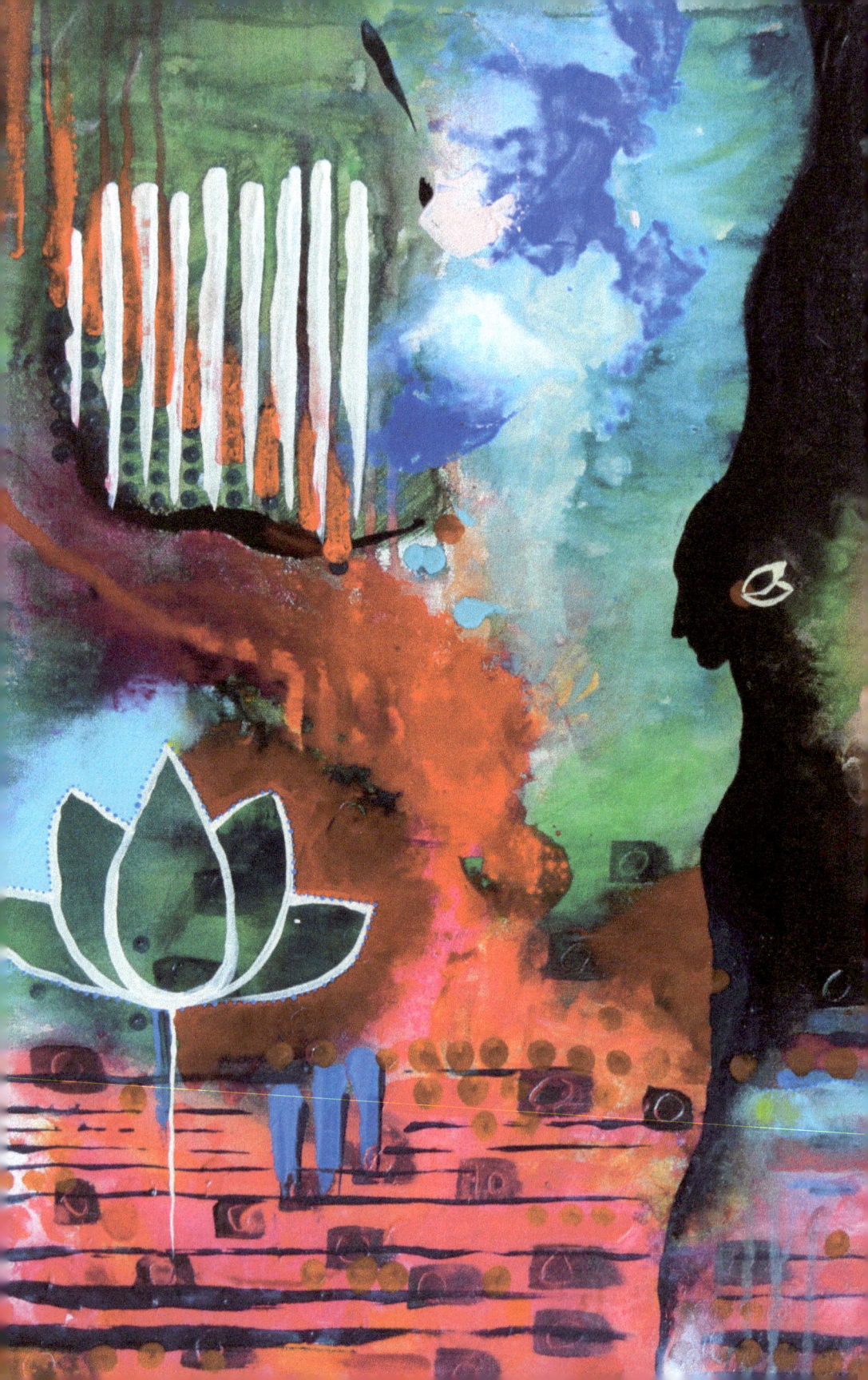

**Al·che·my**
/ˈalkəmē/
*noun*

*The medieval forerunner of chemistry, based on the supposed transformation of matter. A process of liberating something from its fixed physical properties and transforming it into another substance. Ancient alchemists used chemicals and base materials to turn lead into gold.*

**Cre·a·tive Al·che·my**
/krēˈādiv / ˈalkəmē/
*noun*

*The use of art, writing, music, and other creative modalities to alchemize ideas into action, despair into joy, isolation into community. Modern day creative alchemists do not seek to liberate fixed metals. They liberate themselves and others.*

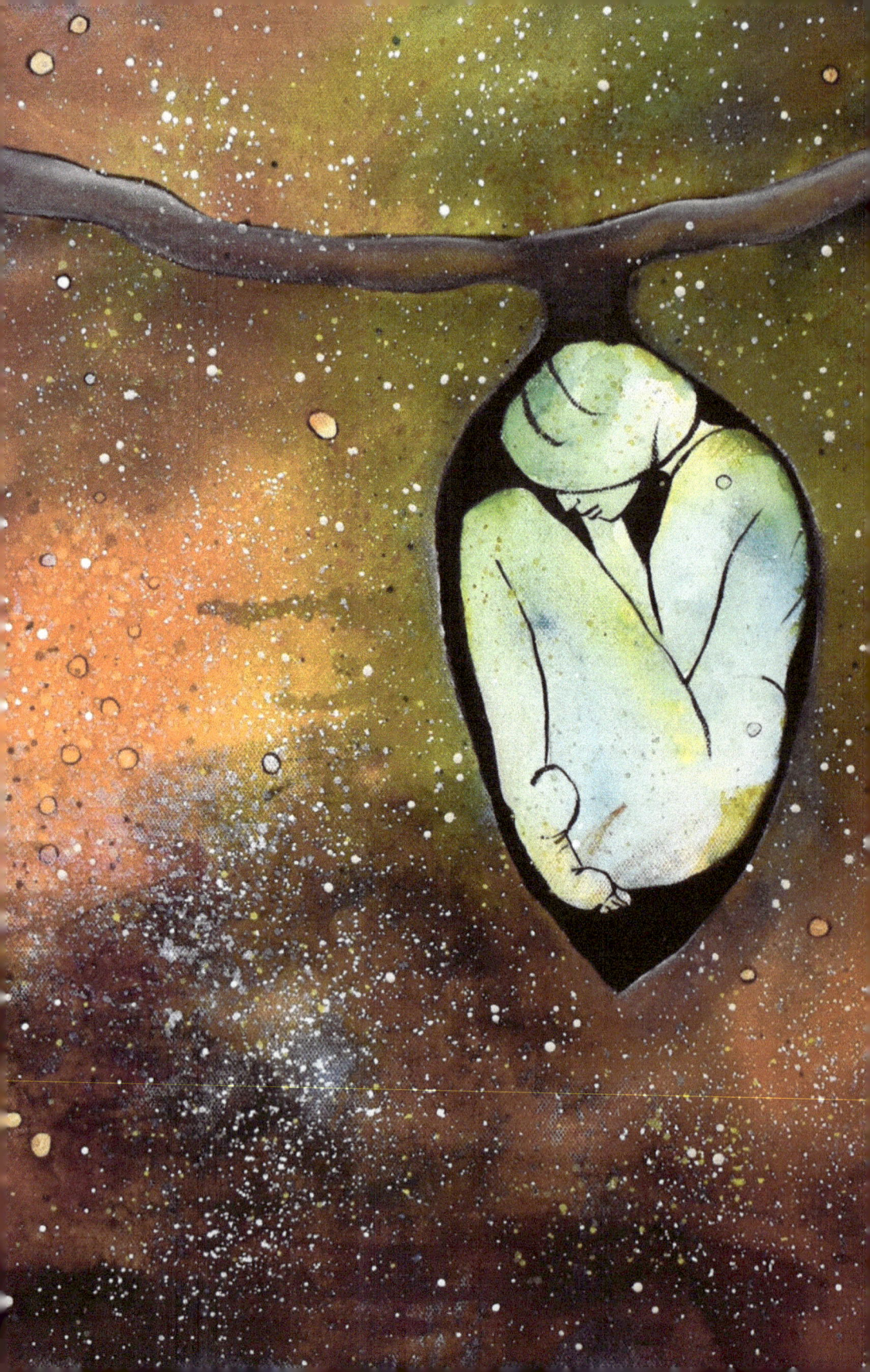

# INVITATION

Once, you were a watery thing.
You, in your dark beginning, lungs full of fluid,
tucked into the pelvis of a person caught dreaming.
Your first decree was to shapeshift,
to perform a miracle of vascular gymnastics:
Breath.

Then your skin, newly exposed to this bright, bold world,
awakened to its own intelligence.
Pressed against warm arms and breast, neck and chest,
a new longing took hold, like a fire in the belly:
Nourishment.

Once satiated, you stretched forth
and unfurled your limbs with a sense of divine urgency.
Someone met your searching hands and held them close.
An inner knowing, born deep in your soft baby bones,
transmitted a signal that lit up your nervous system
and ignited an exploding chain-reaction of neural connectivity:
Belonging.

And although you had no words,
you knew in an instant that you and everything you could perceive
were somehow woven together, a fabric of relationship.
Perhaps a calm rippled across the surface of your face.
Those around you peered into the watery depths of your eyes,
a bottomless sacred well that extended deep into the earth of your
lineage.
The gaze of recognition aroused in you a new iteration of experience:
Joy. Joy. Joy.

~

You began this journey as a shapeshifter — a tuning fork for the transmission of divine information. Everything that followed, from your birth to this moment, has been an experiment in creativity. What you see, how you see it, and the sense-making you craft out of that seeing is called "living." And that, dear one, sums up the creative act.

Here's what I know for sure: this is your one and only precious life on this fragile blue dot. The quality of your hours is the quality of your days is the quality of all the time you have here. Breath, nourishment, belonging, and joy are not negotiable. They are your birthright.

There is no need to hide yourself away or eke out your gifts in small digestible bits. Hit us with your wholeness. Who are you saving it for? My advice? Spend it all. Give it away. Live out loud. And for goodness sake, don't compare the gifts you were given to the gifts of those around you. If we are to survive this life and create a thriving future for those yet to come, we need every last one of us to deliver our gifts into the world and help each other get free.

*The Creative Alchemy Cycle* is a celebration of your creative work in the world. Use this book as fuel. Burn it up and let the exhaust propel you forward.

Do not be afraid.
You already have everything you need to begin.

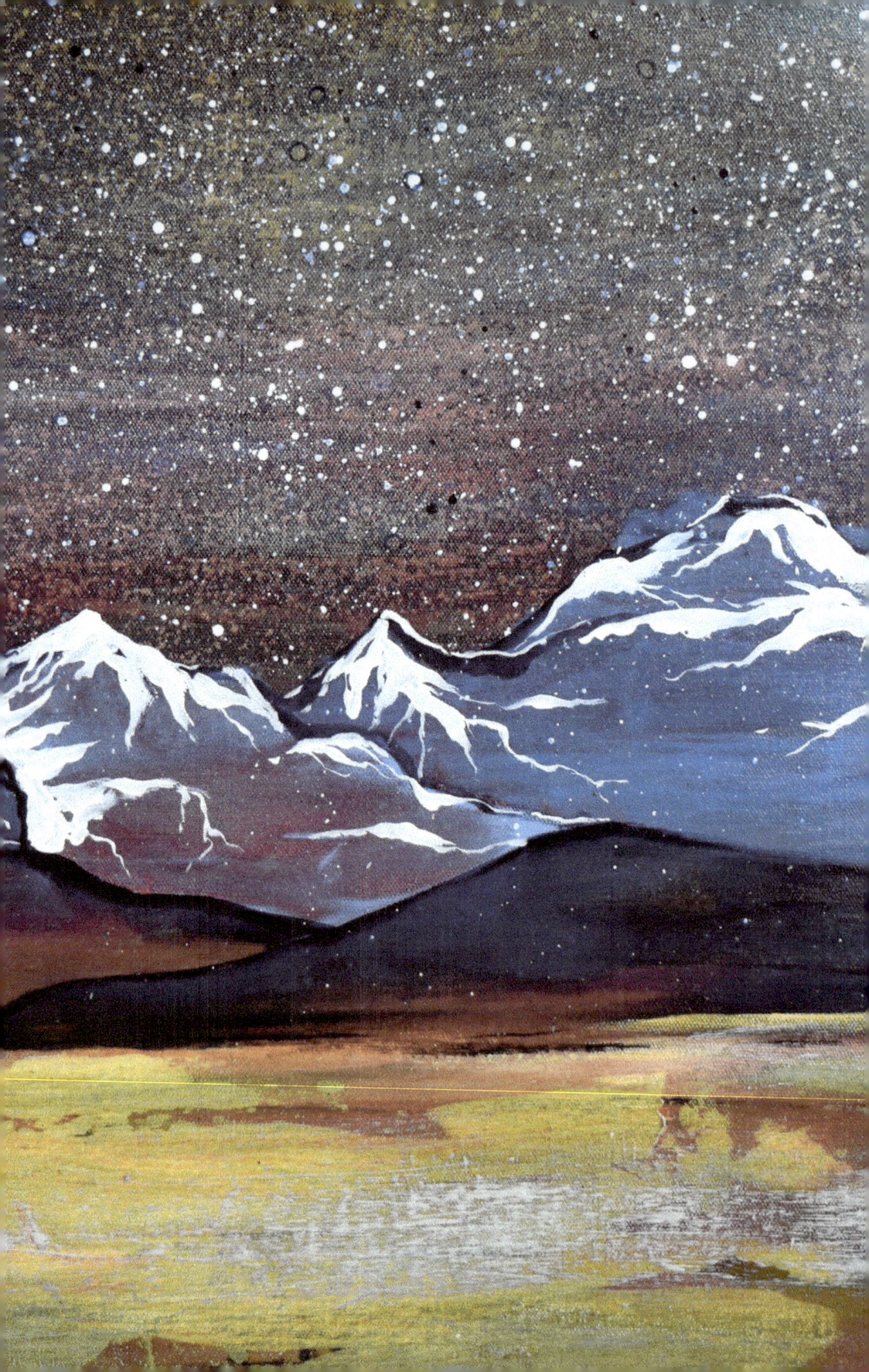

# INTRODUCTION

SMOKE HANGS HEAVY IN THE AIR. THE WALLOWA MOUNTAINS OF Northeastern Oregon, which stand at nearly 10,000 feet to the west and are usually the most prominent visual feature of Pine Valley, are invisible today. It is late August as I write this and Oregon is experiencing its largest fire season in recorded history. The smoke is oppressive, but from my studio window, I can still make out the shape of the Douglas fir that stands at the corner of the fence line.

My home's previous owner, Earl Thompson, planted this tree sometime in the mid-1940's. Earl is long dead now, but I like to think that planting this pine at the end of the second world war was an act of hope for a sustainable future he held in his mind's eye. It turns out that Earl's intentions were less altruistic. His daughter, now in her 80's, tells me that her dad purchased the seedlings from a friend, thinking that they were Juniper. He was hoping to create a little separation from his neighbors with a privacy screen. Instead, he ended up with a row of towering pines planted far too close for comfort.

As I look out upon Earl's pine hedge, the sun continues to rise and a curtain of smoke takes on a rust-orange hue. The era of the mega-fire is clearly underway and I'm fighting the urge to cry. The Douglas fir and I look at each other through the glass. She seems to say, "We were made for these times." She has been here year after year while the Earth spins forward, offering her patterns and lifeways as a blueprint for living, managing water and wind, fluctuations and fire.

I step outside my studio door. Every living thing around me is yellow and sunburned. I walk across the dry, crunchy grass to the tree. It's hot and her gray bark is secreting milky pink sap. I put my hands on her deeply veined skin and wiggle my bare toes into the dusty earth around her roots. For a moment, we breathe together. I close my eyes and repeat her wisdom, "We were made for these times."

~

I live in Pine Valley, a cornucopia-shaped bowl at the base of the Wallowa Whitman mountain range in far Eastern Oregon. Our valley marks the first blush of conifers after traversing east through the high, sagebrush covered deserts of Harney, Malheur, and Baker counties. The trees here are proud, oasis-like creatures that rise in the sky like buildings in a city. They have their own songs, particular to their shape and layout. You can hear them when the breeze comes sliding down through the valley at night. These trees are a border-community, standing sentinel at the edge of the desert, a mix of drought and stream, dust and moss. They are both vulnerable and wildly resilient.

I've been in community with this forest since 2005, but even in that short span of time, I've observed numerous changes, small and large, due to climate fluctuations. This new era of extreme drought combined with soaring temperatures is an imminent threat to this ancient place. Even now, with my hands pressed against Earl Thompson's would-be Juniper turned Doug fir, I can feel her powerful capacity to heal and renew herself. Surely, there is something ancestral and sacred here.

~

How do we manage and make sense of a rapidly changing world and climate? The news cycle peppers us with daily signs of catastrophe, injustice, and ecocide. It is hard to know how to respond or offer alternatives for new ways of engaging.

*The Creative Alchemy Cycle* was born out of my longing for another way forward that centers creativity as a tool for transformation. Olivia Laing best describes this longing in her book *Funny Weather*. She writes, "What I wanted most, apart from a different timeline, was a different time frame, in which it might be possible to feel and to think, to process the intense emotional impact of the news, and to consider how to react, even perhaps to imagine other ways of being. The stopped time of a painting, say, or the drawn-out minutes and compressed years of a novel, in which it is possible to see patterns and consequences that are otherwise invisible." The *Cycle* is a way of tuning our creative process to the rhythm of nature and mirroring Earth's instinct for healing and regeneration. It is a way of making invisible patterns and consequences more visceral and tangible. The inquiry I offer in these pages invites us to intentionally hone our creative impulses with a focus on justice, right-relationship, and personal innovation. It's a homecoming.

The *Cycle* is also a response to an inner question I've been carrying my entire adult life: What is mine to do? (My friend and author Tracy Brown was the first person who helped me to articulate this question in this particular way.) As an avid journal keeper, I have dedicated volumes of writing to this inquiry. And while the answer shifts depending on context and need, it's always rooted in creativity and right-relationship.

My highest hope for this work (the big juicy dream) is two-fold. I want us to share our creative gifts with the larger community and build pathways for collective action and healing on behalf of the greater good. And I want us to experience profound joy and relish earthly delights. After all, what is justice without joy? What is healing without wholeness?

On the surface this process looks like invitations for spending time in nature, creative tutorials, and journal prompts. But as you dive deeper, it manifests as nurturing deep respect for land, developing new ways of perceiving, and strengthening our capacity for empathy, accountability, and creative risk. I want you to treat your thoughts and creative impulses like they matter. Because they do.

For me, creative work is not separate from my life and my living.

It's all interconnected. *The Creative Alchemy Cycle* honors this truth: that you cannot engage with the world and remain separate from it. Just ask my companion, the Douglas fir. Here she is, doing the creative work she was born to do: photosynthesizing, respiring, and regenerating. She is complete unto herself and yet in constant relationship with every other living thing. And it's not simply that the tree is making my life possible in a theoretical way, but rather the tree and I are fused. The *Cycle* helps me make the leap from the myth of each living thing as a discrete self to the truth of our interconnectedness. Not tree *and* me. But tree *as* me.

I believe that we are not here to overcome or fix anything. We are here for joyful adaptation — expanding our resilience, tapping our innate creativity (we all have it), and discovering what might be possible as we meet the challenges ahead. The *Cycle* is how I show up whole and stay in relationship with the people around me and the land I call home. It's also how I slow down, return to my body, engage my creative mind, heal in community, practice accountability, and center nature as my guide in this ever-accelerating world.

And to be clear, the process I offer here is not blind hope or silver-lining-style optimism. It is a way to develop our capacity for uncertainty while centering joy, justice, creativity, mutual care, and community.

As an artist who is committed to collective liberation, it is my greatest pleasure and joy to share this process with you here. My vision for this work is that as we deepen our experience of Earth's creative flow and allow it to inform our own natural rhythms, we'll discover new ways of being, seeing, and taking informed action on behalf of our wellbeing as a people and planet.

In her book *Braiding Sweetgrass*, Robin Wall Kimmerer writes, "It was through her actions of reciprocity, the give and take with the land, that the original immigrant became indigenous. For all of us, becoming indigenous to a place means living as if your children's future mattered, to take care of the land as if our lives, both material and spiritual, depended on it." We all have the capacity to, as Kimmerer states, become indigenous to a place. The *Cycle* has been my way of remembering myself home and waking up to my own indigeneity.

I come from a Gaelic lineage, meaning an ethno-linguistic culture from Scotland, Ireland and Wales. My paternal line immigrated to the United States from 1760 into the 1800s during the Clearances when some 150,000 Scots were removed from their ancestral lands by force and starvation. My maternal line shows up in the U.S. from Ireland during the 1850s, due to famine caused by the potato blight.

My Celtic ancestors knew and understood the sacred interrelated nature of all things and their religious structures, both pagan and Christian, were rooted in human creativity as an expression of the divine imagination. Theirs was a bardic tradition that infused their very stories with sacred information they'd learned from the living Earth. Both their spiritual and creative practices honored the annual cycle of seasonal festivals consisting of the year's chief solar events (solstices and equinoxes) and the midpoints between them.

I've woven the Celtic calendar into the fabric of *The Creative Alchemy Cycle* as a way of calling forth my own ancestral wisdom. But you don't need to be rooted in or even familiar with Celtic traditions to engage with this work. This book will help you connect more deeply with your own cultural and creative practices. We are all interpreters of our past, making new choices about how we will engage with the challenges that lie before us. Our ancestors, whether chosen or by birth, are a profound source of inner intelligence as we build emergent pathways into the future.

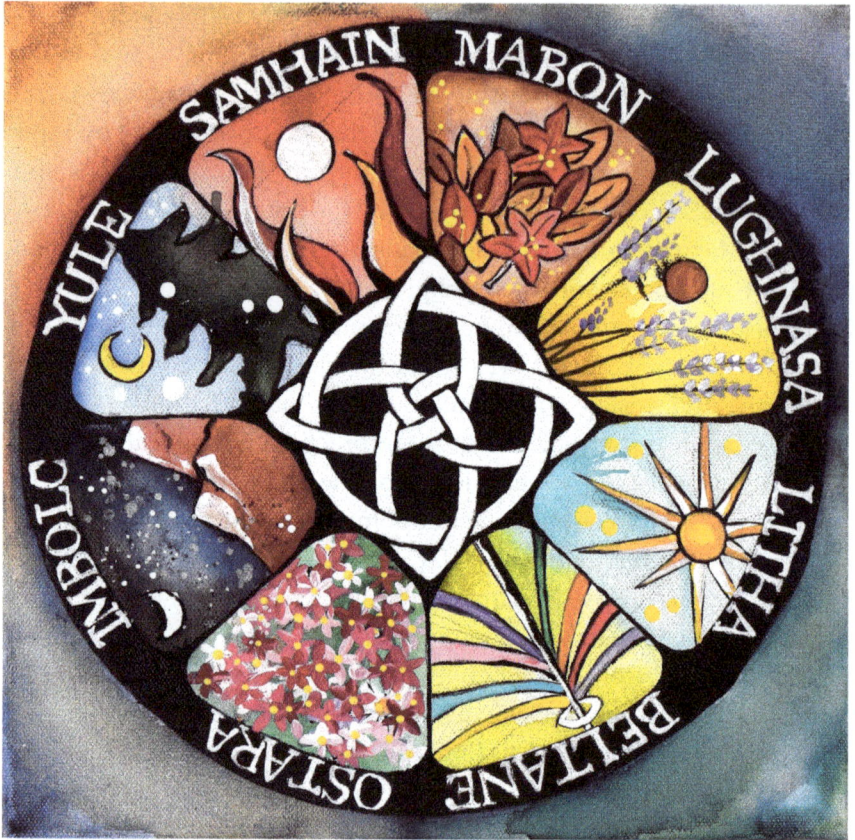

## How to Use This Book

In this book, I share a cyclical creative journey that moves through eight distinct, yet interconnected practices. Each of them serves as a lens through which we may cultivate our creative work and understand the nature of our creative gifts. Each lens corresponds with one of the eight holidays on the Celtic Wheel of the Year.

- Imbolc: Journal Practice
- Ostara: Sketchbook Practice
- Beltane: Embodiment Practice
- Litha: Activist Practice
- Lughnasa: Accountability Practice
- Mabon: Gratitude Practice
- Samhain: Grief Practice
- Yule: Joy Practice

Each of the eight seasonal chapters follows this framework:

**Calling You Home:** A seasonal story in the form of a homily that intertwines my own lived experience with the myths and symbols of each season. These funny, vulnerable, and uplifting stories were created as an active practice, using the Wheel of the Year as a guide. Please enjoy them as a model for your own word-weaving.

**Tend the Altar:** This section welcomes us into a practice of deep noticing and radical listening. Let's get outside and fill our cup. This is our chance to expand, think big, and absorb the beauty and wonder of the natural world, wherever we live. This is where I'll share stories from the landscape of my home in Eastern Oregon as a means of exploring creative inception, inspiration, and the profound wisdom of wild spaces.

**Practices:** The prompts included throughout this book are invitations to gather up our everyday experiences as key ingredients for creative alchemy. These prompts are a vital part of how we'll shape the year before us and show up whole to our work. Plus, they're downright joyful.

The prompts are divided into three sections: Incubation, Action, and Integration. This framework follows what we understand in Celtic culture as the three cauldrons, a kind of Irish chakra system. In Gaelic they are known as the *Coire Goiriath* (Cauldron of Warming or Incubation), the *Coire Ernmae* (Cauldron of Action or Vocation), and the *Coire Sois* (Cauldron of Inspiration or Knowledge).

| Incubation | Action | Integration |
|---|---|---|
| The Earth | The Sea | The Sky |
| The Self | Immediate Circle | The Collective |
| Maiden | Mother | Crone |
| | | |
| Deep Noticing | Embodiment | Alignment |
| Attention | Vocation | Wisdom/Knowledge |
| Self-Interrogation | Choice-Making | Collective Liberation |
| Reflection | Experimentation | Interconnection |
| Excavation | Motion | Inspiration |

**Cross the Threshold:** Observing liminal periods of seasonal transition are a potent part of living in rhythm with Earth's natural cycles. This final section of each chapter offers a bookend to the homily, an epilogue that highlights opportunities to integrate our creative practice into the wider web of community building and social activism.

∾

Lay your hands on the bark of your life. Wiggle your toes in the dust of your experience. Now more than ever, the world needs creative minds, rooted in curiosity, with clear, expressive voices, connected to purpose, who trust, deeply, what they know, feel and see.

This is how we shift culture.

Wherever you are on your creative path and whatever experience you bring to this moment, *The Creative Alchemy Cycle* welcomes you into community. You may be in a fallow period or one of great productivity. You may feel uncertain of your voice or you may know exactly what you want to say. You may find that your purpose is buried or you might be fully centered in your personal mission. You may not yet know how to express the inner workings of your heart or you might be the poet laureate. Either way, you are still a seeker, finding your way, however clear or unclear it may be at this moment.

My ultimate hope is that we can all use the *Cycle* as a way to connect, share, and recognize our collective divinity. Is that too much to ask of a book? Probably. But I am using every tool at my disposal to dismantle the illusion of our separateness.

This home, this Earth, this mother was not made for us alone. We were made together and for each other. Our co-arising was and is the magic of our existence. I am reminded of this fact every time I look up from my little life and see beloved community at the door (that's you!) Mutual care, compassion, and justice-centered stewardship are what matter most now.

I believe that we are the compassionate and creative citizenry that we've been waiting for, unafraid to dismantle old structures, and envision a new future. The most widespread and readily available resource for this transformation is our collective radical imagination. This is why I say that your creativity is a gift. It is a bone-deep tool for healing, justice, and collective liberation. We're all possibility brokers and the creative life is our training ground.

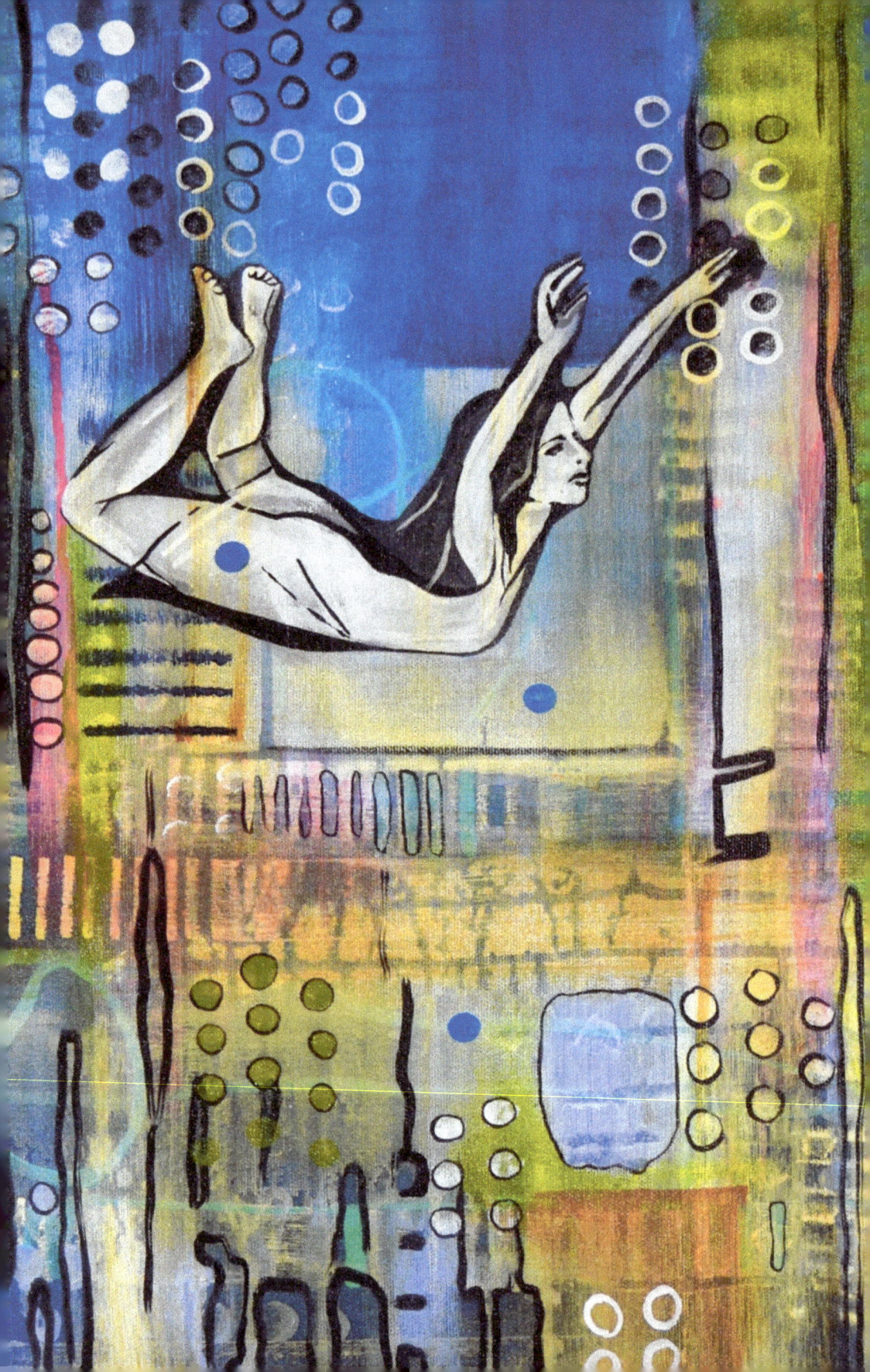

---

# CREATIVITY

## IT'S NOT WHAT YOU THINK IT IS

I LOVE ART. IT'S ONE OF MY FAVORITE THINGS IN THE WHOLE WIDE WORLD. But even more than art, I love creativity. Art is the painting, the play, the quartet, the quilt, the poem, and the product. But creativity is the process, the pathway, the movement, the moment, the curiosity, and the call. For some, creativity is a scary word. It implies that there will eventually be something to show for your time and effort. Probably something called art. I propose that while making art definitely requires creativity, creativity does not mean that art is the automatic end result. Creativity is a way of being present in an ever-changing world, honoring our relationship to that world, and to make meaning from what we notice about that relationship.

This book is about creativity. Not art.

～

One of the first dreams I remember having as a child was of swimming in the Pacific Ocean. This would have been a normal thing to dream because I spent entire swaths of my childhood on the beach in Cayucos, California. In the dream I am shoulder deep in sea water, happily dunking my head under each new wave that approaches. I hear my father call my name from the shoreline. "Sarah, it's time to come in," he shouts. I don't want to return.. My skin has acclimated to the cold water and I am enjoying the kick and flow of my own body. He calls again, this time with more energy.

A large swell grows closer to me and as it nears, I can see that it is much larger than the previous waves. As it crests, the light of the sun shines green and gold through the wave. It crashes over my head and drags me under. I open my eyes but cannot see through the roiling sand and curls of yellow seafoam. In my dream, I realize I'm drowning and I begin to panic. The moment before seawater fills my lungs, I feel my gangly, fighting limbs become smooth along the sides of my body. My legs fuse together into a thick warm tail, and my eyes adjust to the saltwater. I am a sea lion. Slick fur surrounds my body and my nose is twitching with an influx of new scents. I kick free of the undertow and swim away from the shore into the dark open sea. And in my dream I remember feeling a short moment of grief, knowing that I'll never see my family again. But I also felt profound relief to finally be home in my own skin.

As a child, I shared this dream with my Grandma Jane. I was sure that if anyone in the family could unlock the meaning of my dream, it was her. Grandma Jane was a soft-bodied, mischievous woman who loved ice cream, stories, tennis, and her piano. We met together in her sewing room, which was where she kept costumes, books, and gaudy jewelry. But most importantly, it was where we could talk real talk. After I told her of my dream, she fished a book out from under her bed and laid it on her chenille bedspread. I don't remember the title, but on the cover was a group of mermaids dragging a pretty man into the water. She flipped through the book until she found the page she was seeking.

"Here it is. The Selkie!" she said. "This is a very old Celtic story, Sarah. The seal sheds her skin to become a woman and must someday return to the sea. It's Scottish folklore!" She emphasized the word "Scottish" to let me know that I should be proud of our ancestry. I had received a message from somewhere deep in our lineage. Grandma Jane explained that, like the Selkie, I was a person who could move between worlds. The conscious, logical realm of my father on the shore and the subconscious, more mystical realm of the sea. More importantly, the dream showed me I could transform.

～

Over the years, I've understood the Selkie dream to be a metaphor for my creative life. It's a dream about process. Creativity is a shape-shifting tool that calls me to release what has been and swim towards what could be. Creativity is a bridge that connects *what* I do to *how* I do it. The "what" can be anything, truly. But the "how" is creativity. It's what I choose to wear, how I lay out the furniture in my bedroom, how I cook my food, and plant my garden. Whether I'm arranging magnets on my refrigerator or developing a five-year financial plan, I am making creative choices that affect the quality of my day and establish my sense of self in the world. Creativity is how I take action, which is why it lies at the root of my capacity for change-making.

I have always been a creative person. It was recognized in me by my family, nurtured as part of my upbringing, and held sacred by those I shared it with. As a kid, this manifested in many ways. If I was plinking around on a piano, someone would show me a chord. If I admired a sweater, someone would locate a crochet hook and show me how to make a chain of loops. If I became curious about a place, someone would take the time to point me towards a map. The adults in my life rewarded my expressions of curiosity by providing a first step towards learning more. They did not do it for me, nor were they experts in any of these areas of interest. They simply said yes to my creative impulses and put the tools in my hands.

In this sense, I have been very lucky. Centering creativity and highlighting its presence as a daily practice allowed me to weave it into all areas of my life and work. Creativity is like breathing to me. It's as if creativity is a system in the body akin to the circulatory system, the lymphatic system, or the nervous system. And if I don't feed that system, it can't do its right and proper work of keeping me healthy, connected, and thriving.

But I know this is not true for everyone. For many of us, our creative impulse is tied up with ideas about perfectionism, worthiness, and approval. Some of us are still learning to create in the face of doubt and fear, or to identify our unique forms of expression and exploration as creativity. All humans are innately creative and yet there are myriad things that might interfere with natural impulses. If this describes you, then please know that *The Creative Alchemy Cycle* is a permissive and gentle place to practice the slow and steady reclamation of your creativity. Working at a pace that invites deep noticing and reflection is how we come back into right-relationship with our creative gifts and the world around us.

For those of you who are thinking, "Yeah, this all sounds good, but I'm just not creative," I invite you to pause and recognize that you are inadvertently perpetuating a myth that people are somehow exempt from their innate creative gifts.

Think back to when you were a child. Did you ever talk to a plant, or a rock, or a flower? Did you ever turn your lunchbox into a bird's nest? Did you ever find another use for your dinner plate—a frisbee, perhaps? Did you ever locate a tool and use it for something it was never designed for? Did you ever pretend you were someone else or make believe you were an animal? Did you devise a way to fool your siblings into thinking something was true or untrue? Did you ever build something without following the instructions? Then you, my love, are a creative being. No ifs ands or buts.

Astrologer and author Chani Nicholas writes, "To deny my power is to inhibit a whole host of realities from existing in the world. It's not my place to curb the creative possibilities that want to move through me." Chani asks that we recognize the potency of our creative capacities without watering them down or refuting their urgency.

Today, let's hold our doubts and fears lovingly in our hands, and thank them for protecting us. Then let's set them down in a cozy place alongside our path and ask them to wait until we return. After all, their services are no longer needed here. We can always come back for them (or not).

Now that our hands are free, let's consider what we might pick up in place of the doubts and fears we've been carrying! Perhaps a pen? A paintbrush? A needle and thread? A bundle of dried flowers? Let's also consider what we might need along our creative journey. We will be using the Celtic Wheel of the Year to pace ourselves as we move through the seasons ahead. It's also important to note here that you can pick up this book and begin the process at any time during the year. Time is ours and nothing need be rushed. Our creative work will take us outside to commune with the natural world that surrounds us and also find us inside, puttering away in whatever place we call home.

If you're like me, you'll use this book as permission to collect and seek out a variety of materials, supporting a trip to a bead shop, or enabling your indoor plant collection, encouraging your artsy clothing acquisitions, or affirming your sneaky art supply habit. But this is not necessary. Do not load up on materials you'll never use. Rather, let expanding curiosity be your guide. All you need to begin this journey is a journal of some kind and something to write with. That's it. Truly. A journal, a pen, and a receptive spirit will get you everywhere you want to go as a Creative Alchemist.

~

## In Praise of Amateurism

Amateur is one of my favorite words. Unfortunately, it's taken on a negative connotation in the past century, often used as a pejorative for someone who is inept or unskilled. I would like to reclaim the word *amateur* and re-endow it with its original meaning. Amateur has various root meanings. In Latin it stems from *amāre*, which means to love. In French, it means "lover of". There's also a case to be made for the Sanskrit word ámīti, which means to take hold of, grasp, or understand. So to be an amateur means to take hold of or understand something you love. How beautiful!

Many years ago, I spent a holiday season at the Geva Theatre in Rochester, New York. It was during one of their productions of *A Christmas Carol*. Since most of us were away from family, the acting company decided to host a potluck feast in one of the standard issue apartments used to house out of town artists.

After dinner, the actor playing Mrs. Cratchit, Kaia Monroe, pulled out a beat up case covered in travel stickers. She opened it and took out a saxophone. While assembling the mouthpiece and reed, Kaia addressed the group. "I am a proud amateur saxophonist," she said, "and tonight I would like to play for you. I don't think you have to be perfect at something to share it with others. And I think we need to bring back the evening family sing-along. So let's celebrate our amateurism!"

The group circled up around the saxophone with our hot toddies in hand. It was just like Jo March and all of her sisters in *Little Women*. They'd all sit around the piano and sing and play their creaky instruments as a way of entertaining each other on those dark, cold Concord evenings. While Mrs. Cratchit played her best jazzy version of "Oh Holy Night," we smiled and sang and remembered why we loved the arts in the first place. Sure, the arts are entertaining. Sure, it's good to learn new things. But mostly, I think it has something to do with joy.

I want to disrupt this idea that you have to be excellent at something to enjoy it. And I am especially interested in disrupting the notion that if you are good at it, you have to monetize it in some way. *The Creative Alchemy Cycle* is a place to welcome your creative impulses and invite them to join the circle. Let's use our love of art and our joy in the process to expand our sense of what is possible. We will not be perfect. It's going to get messy. The saxophone will squeak. But we will be joyful. And we will take up space and honor our creativity. And in doing so, our creativity will be a catalyst for connection and community building.

∼

Author and activist Joanna Macy says that, "to be alive in this beautiful, self-organizing universe — to participate in the dance of life with senses to perceive it, lungs that breathe it, organs that draw nourishment from it — is a wonder beyond words." There are so many ways to move through the precious hours and days we have on Earth. Joanna Macy reminds us that it's all a gift. And our creative lives are the connective tissue that allow us to make meaning of this "wonder beyond words."

So let's wade into the water, allow the waves to take us out to sea, and invite some playful transformation.

Creativity isn't the cure for everything.
*Creativity is the source of everything.*

Creativity isn't an antidote to grief.
*Creativity is a way to process grief.*

Creativity isn't a painting or a play.
*Creativity is a path and a way.*

Creativity isn't reserved for artists.
*Creativity is a birthright for all.*

Creativity isn't exclusive.
*Creativity is permission.*

Creativity isn't prescribed.
*Creativity is liberatory.*
*Creativity is activist.*
*Creativity is lift-off.*
*Creativity is life.*

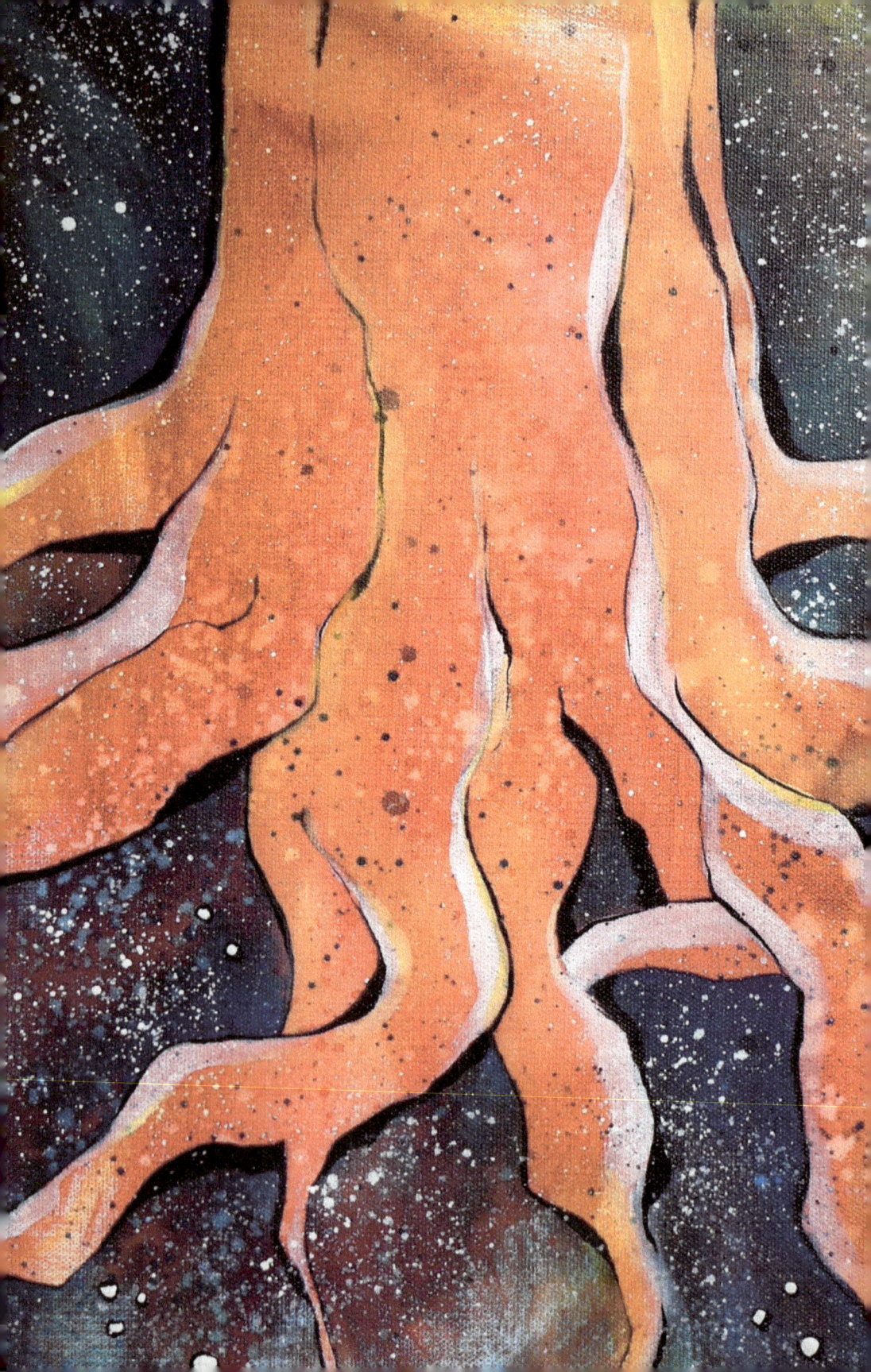

# 2

# WE ARE ROOTS: IMBOLC

## JOURNAL PRACTICE

**The Call:** Your story matters.

**The Question:** What is longing to be born in me?

**The Time:** February 1st and 2nd

**The Origin:** Imbolc (pronounced IM-BLK), also called Brigid's Day, is a traditional Celtic fire festival marking the halfway point between the winter solstice and the spring equinox. The word Imbolc translates as "in the belly" or "in milk."

**The Imagery:** Roots, Birth, Hearth

**The Themes:** Creative Gestation, Incubation, Awakening, and Emergence

WE'RE AT THE BEGINNING AGAIN, FRIENDS. THE EMERGING NEW YEAR invites us to put our ear to the ground and listen for movement beneath the surface. Roots are growing on some of our big ideas. This is quiet, gestational, underground, birth work. We sense that something sacred is on its way. But all things in their own time, yes? Over the next six weeks, we'll take our cues from mother nature and work with potent themes of birth and emergence. We'll honor our creative impulses and unearth buried stories by establishing a journal practice. Gentle invitations for exploration are seeded throughout this chapter that coax our creative vision to take root and grow. The days between Imbolc and the Spring Equinox usher in a time of profound creative germination and growth. It's time to celebrate the unstoppable and insatiable nature of our own life force. Let's get ready to push.

CALLING YOU HOME — A SEASONAL HOMILY FOR IMBOLC

Last week, I drove by a stand of cottonwood trees and noticed three bald eagles sitting patiently in the upper limbs. Their heads were turned in the direction of a snow-covered field, littered with cattle. The birds were still and attentive. Waiting. Imbolc marks the beginning of calving season. After a long winter, the birds were looking for nourishment and it turns out that a cow's afterbirth is an excellent source of iron and protein. Blech. Still, the eagles are a nice perk.

Everything seems expectant now, and only slightly visible if at all, like the gentle curve of a 'just-showing' pregnancy. Whatever your experience of winter, whether it's the ice and snow of Central Maine or the Santa Ana winds of Southern California, Imbolc is a holiday that highlights new life. Just below winter's cold crust, the soil is alive with microbes, and root systems are coming to life as the days lengthen and the sunlight comes on strong.

Imbolc also honors the Goddess Brigid, a midwife deity to the Irish people. Her element is fire and she works as a creative alchemist, overseeing the work of blacksmiths, brewers, bards, birthers, and other creative souls.

I used to work as a doula and postpartum clinician at a birth center in Dallas, Texas. Each time I prepared the birthing suite, I would offer an invocation to Brigid in honor of the act of creation about to transpire. I remember a couple from Austin, Shane and Kat, were particularly touched by this gesture. They were what my grandparents would call "groovy."

The couple showed up in labor on a Saturday with an arsenal of candles, musky massage oils, and a beautiful little meditation bowl that made a clear low tone that resonated for minutes after being struck. Kat assembled an altar. Shane requested that our staff honor their wishes for a totally silent birth. Shane handed out little lanyards to our staff with notepads suspended at the end so we could forgo speaking and instead write on the pads. The birth center was a pretty permissive place, so we agreed, with the caveat that we would speak if there was a health concern.

Early labor is a great time for silent-witchy-candle-burning-bell-bonging. But transitional labor, like all creative acts, requires some serious energy. The staff was not surprised, after many hours of labor, that Kat was not loving the silent treatment. She was in a birthing tub and Shane was doing some meditative breathing by her side. Kat's face was twisted up. The red, overheated skin on her chest was covered in raised bumps like strawberry seeds. Her eyes met mine. I scribbled onto my notepad and showed it to her: "Wanna make some noise?"

"Yes, God, please!" she cried.

Shane's eyes popped open. "Honey, honey! Remember what the book said? Babies born into a silent environment have a better chance of..."

Kat interrupted. "I just gotta get out of this tub."

Shane scooted out of the way to find his shirt while the midwife and I helped Kat out of the tub and to the edge of a four-poster bed where Kat instinctively grabbed the corner and squatted down.

Shane scrambled around looking for his camera and said, "Shouldn't we check her to see if it's time?"

The midwife piped up, "Nope. Kat knows it's time."

There was no stopping what was coming. Kat had planned, assembled the altar, prayed to the ancestors, lit the candles, and rang the bells. Then, in a moment of pure magic, she delivered her child into Shane's trembling hands. No camera. No shirt. No obstacles. Just the awe of the moment and the unmistakable sound of new life.

Every culture has a birth Goddess, because every culture needs one. For the Celts, it is Brigid who cradles birthing mothers in the dark of night. She is the Goddess of new beginnings, ruling over the alchemical arts and the mystery of creation. She is Inspiration, Life Giver, and Hearth Tender.

When I delivered my own child, Charlie, it was Brigid who showed up. Something was wrong with my baby. It was Brigid who stood with my midwives when they made the call to transfer Charlie to the NICU. It was Brigid who stayed with me, alone in my bathroom cleaning up the afterbirth. She held me as I held Charlie during his first seizures. And she steadied my hands when I gave Charlie his first doses of Phenobarbital. It was then that I realized Brigid does not promise healthy children. What she offers is creative allyship.

Creation is messy and rarely follows the trajectory we think it will. Imbolc asks us to have faith and tend our creative fires. Brigid will be there to help us when we pull the iron from the fire, thrust it into the ice-cold water and see what we've wrought.

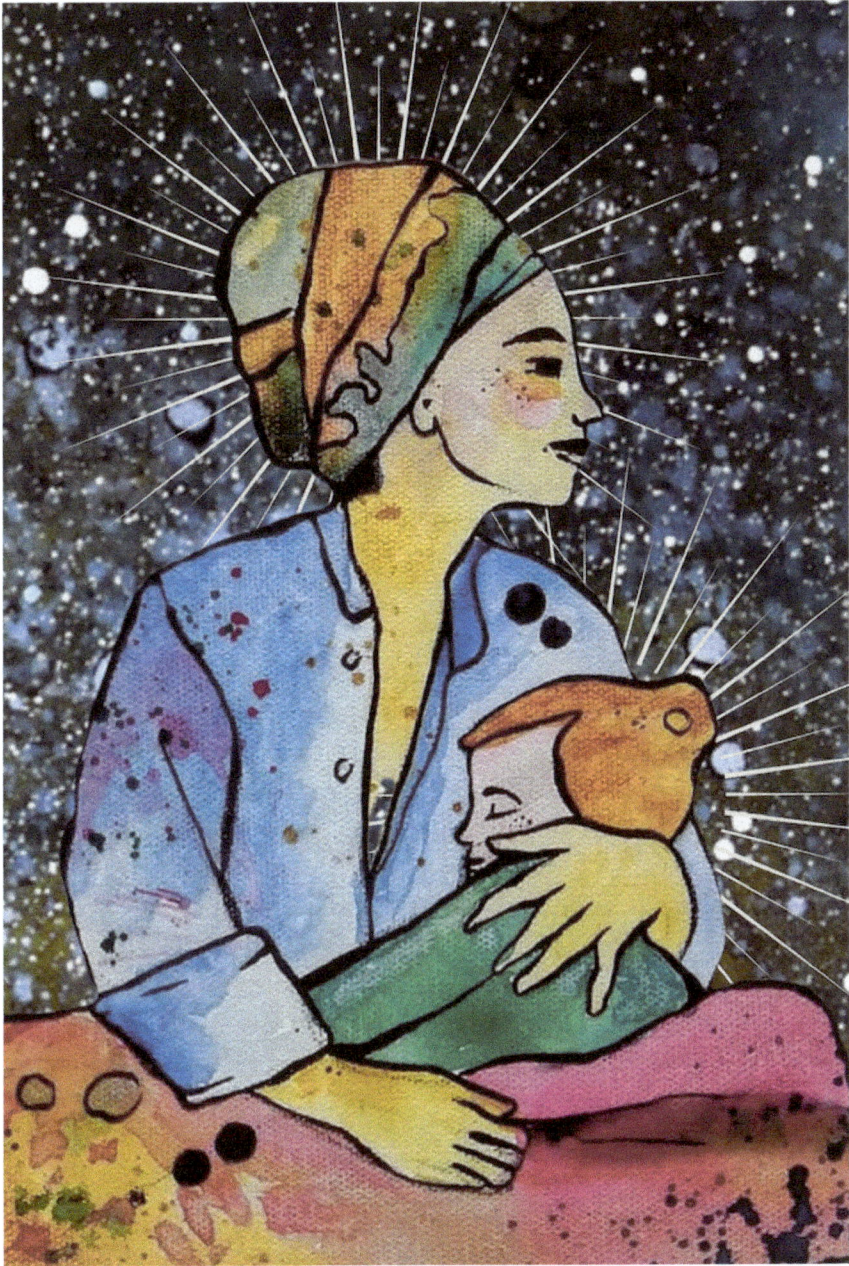

## Tend Your Altar

As we move through the Creative Alchemy Cycle, we'll create and tend a variety of altars. For our purposes, an altar is any space where we intentionally ritualize process. Altars are a sacred place to practice reverence, reflection, remembrance, and gratitude. They focus our sense of purpose and also act as a kind of homecoming, calling us back to ourselves.

Altars can be simple, highly curated, or stumbled upon. As we move through the seasons, I'll encourage you to gather natural objects that feel special or important to adorn your altars. Some examples could be rocks, herbs, seeds, feathers, and other found items. You'll also be invited to add personal items like jewelry, pictures, letters, art, fabric, etc. The options are endless. The key is to let your senses lead the way.

During our journey along the Wheel of the Year, we'll be exploring two kinds of altars. The first altar practice will begin in the great wide open. Mother nature has a habit of creating little altars everywhere. It could be a flat rock along the bank of a stream, a sandy expanse at the edge of a lake, a fallen log at the border of a city park, or a spray of roadside poppies. These are places of great potency that call us to pause, practice deep noticing, and offer thanks.

We'll also build and maintain a physical altar that honors you and your creative practice. Your personal altar will likely change with the seasons. It can be assembled on a table, a windowsill, a nightstand, or even outdoors on a stump or tucked away in your garden or front stoop. We'll imbue this sacred space with seasonal intentions and natural ephemera collected from the outdoors.

### Nature's Altar

Let's begin an intentional practice of noticing nature's altars. Today, I walked ten minutes east of my home to Pine Creek, which runs along our valley floor. The cottonwood branches that flanked the waterway were covered in hoarfrost under a soft blanket of fog. Their roots stretched out over the creek, exposed and twisted into braids like Celtic knotwork by the water flow of previous seasons.

I came upon a beaver dam that bridged a narrow section of the creek. What a thrill to stumble upon the creative work of other creatures. I closed my eyes and allowed my shoulders to soften. The moving water made a thin, tin-like murmur as it eddied and sluiced through the expertly woven debris. The cottonwoods framed a table of ice, which formed behind the dam like an altar to honor winter's promise: what is now dormant, will rise again. The snow will melt, the creek will flow, and the sun will reclaim the souls of every living thing.

Nature's altars offer ample inspiration for our creative work. The woven dam, the knotted roots, and the metallic tune of the water, all working together as a kind of place-based art installation. And somewhere, a beaver is tucked deep in their lodge, waiting to emerge from their slumber in time to be nourished by the fruits of their seasonal creative work.

## Personal Altar

Our personal altars are an outward reflection of our creative cycles. Selecting natural objects from our outdoor sojourns for display on our personal altars is a powerful way to make the shifting seasons tangible and build a focal point for our creative work.

Before leaving the dam, I scanned the scene for a memento. My eyes lighted upon a spray of seed pods, covered in frost, waiting for the right moment for resurrection. They had been in this frozen state for the entirety of January. How incredible that these skeletal botanical structures, appearing as though dead, will soon wake up and expand their root systems in search of water in advance of the spring bud-break. And all this before they ever show signs of a come-back above ground — a wild and faithful act of hope at the end of winter.

I knelt down beside the pods. My knee sank into the muck and my denim pants absorbed the snow. The skin on my shin puckered from the cold. I asked a seed pod for permission, listened for an affirmative response, then snapped off its head and tucked it into my coat pocket.

Once home, I pulled the seed pod from my pocket and placed it on my altar. A few seeds escaped their encasement and scattered across the surface of my altar. The pod symbolizes creative quiescence – a potent reminder that, like this seed pod, we are all in a state of quiet readiness.

Imbolc calls upon us to hold the highest vision for our future. Soon the seeds will spill out, the cottonwoods will bud, the ice will thaw, hibernating animals will emerge, and the creek will break water. Creative birth work is Imbolc's calling card and tending an altar is a wonderful way to get intentional about what we want to bring forth.

### Altar Practice

Whether you're a practiced altar keeper or you've never thought to make one, allow this invitation to offer deep permission for playfulness. Begin by taking a breath. Now take a slow stroll around your home. Is there a surface that longs to be adorned with magical objects? Is there a corner or a windowsill that can support a daily pause. Is it both accessible to you and also protected from the natural traffic of your home's inhabitants? Once you've selected a location, wipe down the surface with a cloth and tidy up the area around it. And as you do this, hold this question at front of mind: *What is longing to be born in me?*

Now it's time to assemble a few items for your altar. A traditional Imbolc altar includes a white candle to symbolize your inner fire and a bowl of water, a symbol of Brigid's sacred well. But you can include anything that symbolizes creative fire and new life. An altar becomes especially potent if the items you choose to display are connected to your lineage or your personal life. I like to arrange a candle with some forced spring bulbs, a collection of dried seed pods, and a Celtic Brigid's cross woven from straw. Each object resonates with Imbolc's themes of birth, emergence, and awakening.

Once you've arranged your objects, light your candle and find a comfortable place to sit or stand. Gaze upon the objects. What is longing to be born in you? Which birth Goddess will you call upon as collaborator and creative ally? Perhaps you'd like to call upon your ancestors (human, animal, plant or otherwise) for guidance. Ask them to walk alongside you in the weeks ahead as you explore the natural world around you, excavate your own stories, and kindle your creative fires. When you feel a sense of fullness, close by offering thanks and extinguish your candle. Watch the smoke dissipate and imagine that it is your intention permeating the very air you breathe. And so it is.

JOURNAL PRACTICE

This season, we'll start a journal. And if you're already a devoted journal-keeper, this is an excellent opportunity to deepen your practice. It doesn't matter whether you're writing in a spiral-bound notebook from the dollar store or a leather bound journal that looks like it fell off the bookshelf at Hogwarts. The important thing is that you have lots of space to tell your story.

Your story is compelling because it happened to you. And your story matters because you are not alone in the experience of it. At the same time, it's completely unique to you. Your interiority is a landscape no one on Earth has ever explored. You are the sole traveler. And the act of sharing your story will serve as someone else's roadmap home. But most importantly, it is *your* roadmap home.

Keeping a journal disrupts forgetting. We always think that we'll never forget the surprising, distinct, phenomenal details of our lived experiences. But then the mind works its slippery dark magic and changes what we think we thought we knew, infuses our memory with other narratives, or just completely wipes them away. A journal practice is how we softly catch the elusive butterfly of experience in our hands and sketch it into being before releasing it back to the wide open sky.

A journal practice is the foundational root system for all my creative work. Every play I've ever written, every painting I've ever painted, every story I've ever told, and every workshop I've ever taught started as a granular spark in my journal. Not every spark caught flame, of course. There are a myriad of ideas, pages filled with lists, thoughts, and musings, that were equally valuable without resulting in an "outcome".

I was twelve years old when I received my first journal as a birthday gift from my Grandma Jane. It was a beautiful volume of lined pages, wrapped in dusky rose and mint green chintz fabric. Inside the first page she wrote, "I believe you could write someday, and every good writer keeps a journal. Let this be the first of many journals. Write about all you see, think, feel, or do. It's a wonderful habit."

My grandmother gave me a beautiful introduction to living a creative life and showed me how to develop my own creative identity by keeping a journal. We all deserve this kind of grandmother energy in our life — an elder who is rooting for us, and providing generous resources for our own artistic emergence. If, perhaps, you were not afforded this kind of permission as a child, please let this book serve as permission. My Grandma Jane and I are inviting you to keep a journal and honor your story.

There are many ways for creatives to keep a journal. Some of you will write, while others will keep a photo-log, capture film, blog, create recorded audio files, paint, knit, or collage. The container we are creating here holds space for many methods of personal expression. The possibilities are truly endless.

Whatever your modality, we will be using our journal throughout *The Creative Alchemy Cycle*. It will be our primary tool for creative inception, idea incubation, transformative living, and making meaning. Even if you never share these pages, images, or audio files with another living soul (although I hope that you will), a journal practice is a direct path to creative discovery, which will in turn, affect everything and everyone around you.

## Incubation

It might be helpful to think of journal keeping as conversing with the self. This work is for you and by you. Free writing is an accessible and valuable technique for beginners and professionals alike that involves writing with an open-minded and non-judgemental gaze. No editing needed. I use this technique as a way to capture my ideas and jot them down at the pace in which they occur. It allows me to better understand the world around me, and to think "out loud" on the blank page or canvas.

Before we dive in, here's a question to prime the pump of inspiration and warm ourselves up a bit. If you're just beginning your writing practice, this is a wonderful question with which to christen your journal! And if writing is already a steady friend, allow this prompt to infuse your journal with some fresh delight. Spend as much time as you like free writing with this prompt:

**What does joy mean to me and how does it show up in my life?**

～

In his book, *Consolations: The Solace, Nourishment and Underlying Meaning of Everyday Words*, David Whyte writes, "To feel a full and untrammeled joy is to have become fully generous; to allow ourselves to be joyful is to have walked through the doorway of fear." For our purposes, let's think about joy as a profound and intentional state of being, different from happiness and more akin to awakened. There will be times in the cycle (as in life) when we'll navigate rough waters and dark shadows, but always with an eye towards authentic expression and joyful transformation.

One of the fastest ways to deplete joyful energy is to relegate it to the category of "task." Joy is not a to-do, it's an internal compass. Joy is not a box to check, it's reclaimed grace. To ensure we have access to this foundational birthright, we must cultivate it with intention. Your journal is the perfect place to do that.

Let's take our cue from the brilliant poet and author Ross Gay. In his poem "Sorrow Is Not My Name," he writes, "...there are, on this planet alone, something like two million naturally occurring sweet things, some with names so generous as to kick the steel from my knees: agave, persimmon, stick ball, the purple okra I bought for two bucks at the market. Think of that."

**What tangible, "naturally occurring sweet things... kick the steel from your knees"? List them in your journal. Ross Gay**

**offers agave, persimmon, stick ball, purple okra. Mine right now are coffee with cream, soft snow, salted caramel, and flannel. List the many tangible things that bring you pleasure and joy. Easy joy. Simple joy. Your list can be as long or as short as you like.**

Since the season of Imbolc has us dreaming forward for the year ahead, let's consider the trajectory of our year. We're going to spend some time now on seasonal joys. In your journal, write out each month of the year starting with January and ending with December. Leave some space between each of the twelve months.

**For each month, write two or three delights that are really only available to you during that time of year. These are seasonal joys like cherries from your local orchard in June, the Perseid meteor shower in August, a new season of your favorite TV show in December.**

## Action

The lists above are informative touch points on their own, but let's activate and transform them into a roadmap for the year ahead. This is a process we can do at the beginning of each year as we answer Imbolc's call: What is longing to be born in me?

I call it "Delights to Cultivate" – an annual manifesto of personal delights as an alternative to new year's resolutions. It is also a tangible reminder that joy is my birthright and pleasure need not be separate from my work as a change-maker and artist. (Psst... you're a change-maker and artist too.)

New Year's resolutions always feel like terrible little nagging tasks. They usually represent the things we neglected last year that we drag into the new year to haunt our idle hours. And is it me, or do they always seem to be about not doing something or losing something or stopping something? Lose weight. Quit wasting time. Whoooee — Just thinking about it gives me hives.

**Delights to Cultivate**

We are going to create a list of delights to cultivate in the year to come. These are juicy, joyful everyday acts of pleasure and healing that we want to call into our lives. These are not "to-dos." We have plenty of those already clogging up the arteries of our creative flow. Instead, these are pleasures, pure and simple.

We'll be selecting simple actions and mind frames that call these joys into being. Look back over your previous lists. If one of your "naturally occurring sweet things" is bees, then perhaps that translates into "Celebrate the honey bees that frequent my garden." Make sense?

Here are some examples from my past lists:

Delight: Paint brushes
Write: Place art materials in my daily path as a reminder to play.

Delight: Linen
Write: Delight in the feeling of linen against my skin.

Delight: Quiet home
Write: Observe when moments of peace and silence fill my home and give gratitude.

Delight: Cherries
Write: Savor the taste and texture of fresh cherries.

Delight: Good Conversation
Write: Cultivate deep listening — to people, to my inner workings and to the world around me.

A note to your inner editor: If you find yourself transforming these into "to-dos," resist the urge. Take a breath and remember that 'simple joy' is the star of this show. Here's an example of a re-frame I recently used for one of my own lists. I wrote, "Purge my closet." Then, after a deep breath, I reframed it as, "Relish wearing clothes that represent the real me."

If you'd like to organize your joys according to the calendar of the year and list them seasonally, great. You can also let it be more free form, as I did in the list above. Ready? Set? Go!

When you've completed your "Delights to Cultivate," tack them up somewhere visible where you'll see them every day in the year ahead.

## Integration

Let's broaden our definition of journal keeping to also include handwritten letters. Letters are a dynamic way to build connections and communicate with care and authenticity. This practice moves us out of free-writing and invites us to consider our audience. We can write letters to ourselves directly in our journals or expand the circle and create letters for others.

As a doula, I incorporated letter writing into my work at the birth center. Six weeks after each delivery, I gave the family a letter I'd written to their baby, retelling the story of their birth – a journalistic record of their creative emergence. To share an origin story (or any story) is a powerful form of creative alchemy. It says, "Your story matters." Shane and Kat deeply appreciated this gesture because their birth was such a wild ride, they barely remembered the details. Memory is funny like that.

I propose that we reinvigorate the lost art of letter writing. Letters are a squeal-out-loud-when-they-arrive kind of joy. They make it into my list of "Delights to Cultivate" in some form every year. Their analog nature means that they can be held, treasured, and even lost. You can tuck little goodies inside the envelope — perhaps a pressed flower or a photo. They smell of the hands that held them. Letters are precious, intimate, intentional.

Letter writing is also a mindfulness practice, chiefly because it tunes our creative impulse towards deep noticing. A quick look through your local bookstore and you'll find volumes of literature and research about "mindfulness" that you are free to explore. But for our purposes, I define mindfulness as our ability to be fully present, aware of where we are and what we're doing.

Not only do handwritten letters offer us a mindful creative process, but they foster a deeper connection with friends and family, giving us an active tool for building beloved community. When composed with intention, letters create intimacy and a sense of proximity — not just in the words written on the page, but also in the style of handwriting, the feel of the paper, and the structure of the envelope. They all point to the care and thought given by the sender. They also allow us to share our thoughts in silence without having to say them aloud on a phone or over a video chat. (This was a huge bonus for young Sarah, who wanted to connect about hard stuff sometimes.) I remember writing to a childhood friend during the course of my parents' divorce. She had been through a divorce as well and at 13-years-old, we were able to share some really profound thoughts and emotions via our weekly letters.

Letters create pathways for new ways of perceiving. There is a huge difference in what I write to a friend and what I might text or say over the phone. The things I choose to share and the manner in which I share them are altered by the letter writing process — more expressive than an email or text, more succinct than a sprawling phone conversation. When I write, I'm able to perceive my life with a little more objectivity and depth.

For me, one of the unexpected outcomes of letter writing is that it helped me to cultivate patience. Our lives are so full of instant messages and immediate results. There is a waiting period built into the mechanics of letter writing. Writing a letter means locating paper and pen, sitting down, thinking about what I want to say, and then composing the words to express whatever it is I want to express. I relish this deliberate pace. It is a tangible way to breathe air into my reactivity and process the events of my life at a pace that invites awareness. Focusing my attention to each word and phrase I write allows me to assess what I really think about things — similar to what happens when I journal. It's a slow artform.

So buy some stamps and put pen to paper! Your letters can be simple correspondences with only a few words or a favorite quote.

They can also be quite detailed with pages upon pages of observances, thoughts, and questions. They can even be sketches without any words at all. Let your own intuitive style and mood lead your letter writing practice.

## One-Word Prompts for Imbolc

In the following chapters, I offer a 30-word list for each of the eight Celtic holidays on the Wheel of the Year. You can use these to free-write in your journal, to draw in your sketchbook, or in any other way you like.

Delight • Birth • Root • Hearth • Thaw
Journal • Awaken • Eagle • Resolution • Begin
Letter • Patience • Creation • Incubate • Solace
Ice • Labor • Pace • Frost • Story
Tend • Emerge • Mindful • Mirror • Newborn
Winter • Lover • Foundation • Transform • Dream

## The Next Six Weeks

The time between Imbolc and the spring equinox is roughly six weeks. Let's use this time to write one letter a week. You can write letters directly into your journal or you can send them off to friends. The wonderful thing about a letter is that you can write it to anyone, even to yourself. You can also write letters you may never send or to people who wouldn't be able to receive them. You could write a letter to your six-year-old self. You could write a letter to the Sycamore tree that died last year in your backyard, or an old boyfriend, or a future friend you haven't met yet, or to an ancestor, to a favorite flower, to your grief or to your joy. You can even write to the Goddess Brigid, patron saint of creative endeavor. You can write your letters without structure or you can use the following launch points:

I envision a future where…

I am actively holding space for…

I am preparing for a time when…

CROSS THE THRESHOLD

Winter isn't over. Spring isn't here. I'm feeling restless. My mother calls it "antsy." I am feeling the impulse to rush. I'm noticing my desire for the flower, the bee, the sunlight. But now is not the time. Now is the time for observing, planning, soil tending, and attentive listening.

How do you manage this feeling — this sense of existing between the place where you long to be and the place where you are?

These days, I'm taking my cues from nature. Spring is still many weeks off and those skeletal cottonwoods along the banks of Pine Creek remain unchanged. But I know they're hard at work beneath the surface, readying themselves. They remind me that creative incubation is just as important as the bright, showy blooms of creative fruition. Still, I'm restless for change.

One of the things I love most about maintaining a creative practice in rhythm with nature is that it reveals the brilliance of existing natural patterns. Imbolc, like all of the fire festivals (Beltane, Lughnasa, and Samhain) mark the "in-between" seasons. They are liminal holidays that highlight ecological and energetic transitions as opposed to the equinoxes and solstices, which more broadly mark the culmination of the season.

Our creative practice can then be a way to absorb and apply those natural patterns to our own community building and collective care efforts. Imbolc is a quiet time for dreaming together. Let our work here together be a pathway for this collective becoming.

February's longer days are coaxing the roots awake. So much is happening out of sight, buried deep in the soil. We cannot see it, but tremendous energy is building up just below the surface. We're in a state of faith-time, friends. I can't wait to see what happens next. In the meantime, take care of those around you, make use of the resources at your disposal, take notes in your journal and plan for the coming emergence. Anticipation is half the fun.

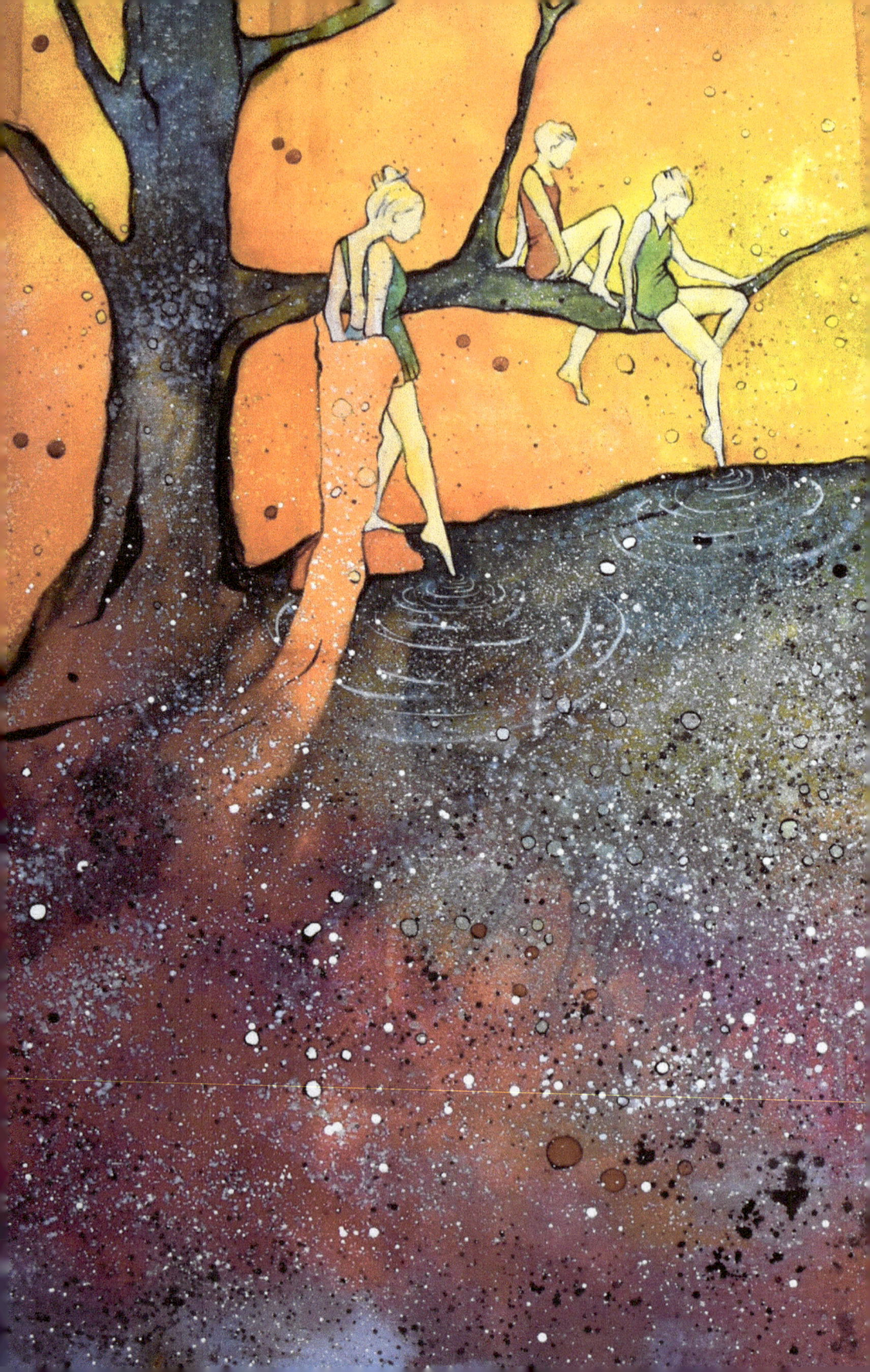

# 3

# WE ARE WATER: OSTARA

## SKETCHBOOK PRACTICE

**The Call:** Trust what you know.

**The Question:** How does inner wisdom flow through me?

**The Time:** March 19th - 21st

**The Origin:** Ostara, also known as the vernal equinox, marks the first day of spring and the halfway point between the solstices. Ostara, also known as Ēostre, is a Germanic goddess of spring and dawn. In Scotland, this day is often called *Alban Eilir,* which translates as "The Light of the Earth."

**The Imagery:** Water, River, Ocean, Stone

**The Themes:** Creative Flow, Perception, Intuition, and Connection

THE VERNAL EQUINOX IS UPON US. BUT THERE'S NO NEED TO ALERT THE plants and animals. They already know. The pheasant, the doe, the mushroom, the mouse. They are spring's eternal partners, co-arising, blinking their eyes open as they inhale the scent of wet earth. Seeds that were once dreaming in the dark have cracked open and pushed their way into the light. Spring's emergent energy is infectious. Do you feel it? After the long dark winter? That corporeal longing to stretch, drink deep, and grow from the inside out? Over the next six weeks, we'll bear witness to Earth's verdant awakening, drink from the sacred well of our creativity, and begin a sketchbook practice. This chapter is a creative laboratory for building our own visual and imagistic vocabulary. We'll draw what we notice and notice what we draw. Ostara is a time to tap the reservoir of our inner knowing, breach the dams of our doubt, and invite our creativity to flow free.

### Calling You Home – A Seasonal Homily for Ostara

I grew up on the central coast of California near the small seaside town of Cayucos. Every year it was the same. The first sunny weekend in March, as the sun crossed from south to north over the celestial equator, our family would hit the beach. And Cayucos was a quick 45 minute drive from my hometown of Paso Robles to the public shoreline — 38 minutes if my dad drove. Cayucos is the Spanish version of a Chumash word for canoe or boat. The Chumash were the original indigenous stewards of the central California coastline and they used to fish the giant kelp beds that thrived just North of current day Cayucos.

The Cayucos of my youth was a quaint and out-of-the-way hamlet with a corner candy store that sold jelly beans and chocolate sea shells. It was a lightly populated place, about 1700 residents according to the 1980 census, and hosted a sand sculpture contest every fourth of July, in which our friend Ray DeMerit would always place. The year I turned eight, he won first prize for a trio of charging buffalo in honor of those he'd seen during a recent trip to the Dakotas. And by nightfall, just like those graceful beasts of the upper Midwest, the high tide swept them away.

My brother Joel and I spent hours on the beach, dragging our lithe bodies over craggy rocks to find sea anemone and hermit crabs. We'd splash around and tie ourselves up with long whips of slimy kelp, and then return to our sandy towels happily exhausted and sunburned.

Year after year, we'd return at the top of the sunny season to swim in the Pacific. By the time we were nine and ten, we were old pros — strong enough to wade into the deep and brave the waves. Sometimes, depending on the moon phase, the waves would really kick up. Surfers from all over San Luis Obispo county would make their way out to the coastline for a shot at the perfect funnel. You don't really understand the silly California exclamation "tubular, dude," until you see the big waves of a full Cayucos moon.

Joel was a talented body surfer. He picked it up so easily. I'd watch him swim hard into a big wave, then at the last minute fold his body into a turn as the wave crashed overhead. He'd disappear for a moment and then, like a piece of driftwood, pop out in front of the seafoam and ride it all the way to the shallows.

"Just try it," he said. "There's really nothing to it. You just pick your wave, feel the rush, straighten your body and keep your head up."

I waited for some time. How would I know which wave to pick?

A small undulation began on the horizon. It was some distance away, so I knew I'd have time to swim out and meet it. I had a strong freestyle crawl stroke and trusted my own power. But as I moved closer to the growing swell, I could feel the water cycle beneath me and pull my body with speed away from the shoreline. I began to panic. My breath became short and I turned to swim back. The wave came on quickly and instead of swimming to the top of the crest like Joel always did, I felt my legs and chest drag down to the trough, which is the bottom-most part of a wave. Then in an instant I was under.

The wave shoved my body to the seafloor and rolled me like a stone. And in my turning, I lost my sense of direction. Churned up with the sand and seaweed, I didn't know which way was up. I threw my arms wide in an attempt to stop the spin and felt my forearm scrape along a rock. The salt stung the open gash and as I choked down an impulse to gasp, my nostrils filled with saltwater and granular bits of sea-stuff. I was drowning.

When I was little, I dreamed of being a Selkie and breathing underwater. And sometimes I imagined that I was part mermaid. In that moment, fighting the rip tide, face shoved into the unforgiving ocean bed, I prayed to transform into some sort of sea lion or gilled creature. I needed oxygen and I needed it now.

Joel grabbed my shoulder and said, "Sarah, you can stand. Just stand up."

The water receded as Joel helped me off my knees to my feet. I coughed up sea water, rubbed the sand from my tear ducts, and told Joel that I hated him for making me want to body surf.

Years later, I stood at his bedside in the Santa Maria hospital after an overdose. I asked, "How can you keep doing this to yourself?"

He said "There's nothing to it. You just pick your wave and feel the rush."

But I knew that eventually he'd forget to keep his head up.

I return as often as I can to the Pacific. If I can't get to Cayucos, I find some other coastal place. It's all the same water. I didn't turn into a mermaid or a sea lion that day, but I did discover the sheer power and elemental potency of the sea. She is part of my inner landscape now, embedded in my every move. It all ends up in my art: the water, the kelp, the grief, and the gravitational pull. I'm a water woman, born with the moon in Cancer, dragged to the bottom of the ocean, tumbled like a rock in the briny waters, shipwrecked, spitting, sputtering, and born again onto dry land.

For me, water is a healer. And at this time of year, the Spring Equinox promises to transform the surrounding snow into life energy. The ice will melt, the creeks will bulge, the rivers will swell, and the sea will call back all her beloved molecules.

Even Joel, whose ashes were cast by my own trembling hands into the bright briny waters of the Pacific, found his way home. I too, will one day breathe underwater and let that undercurrent sweep me out to sea.

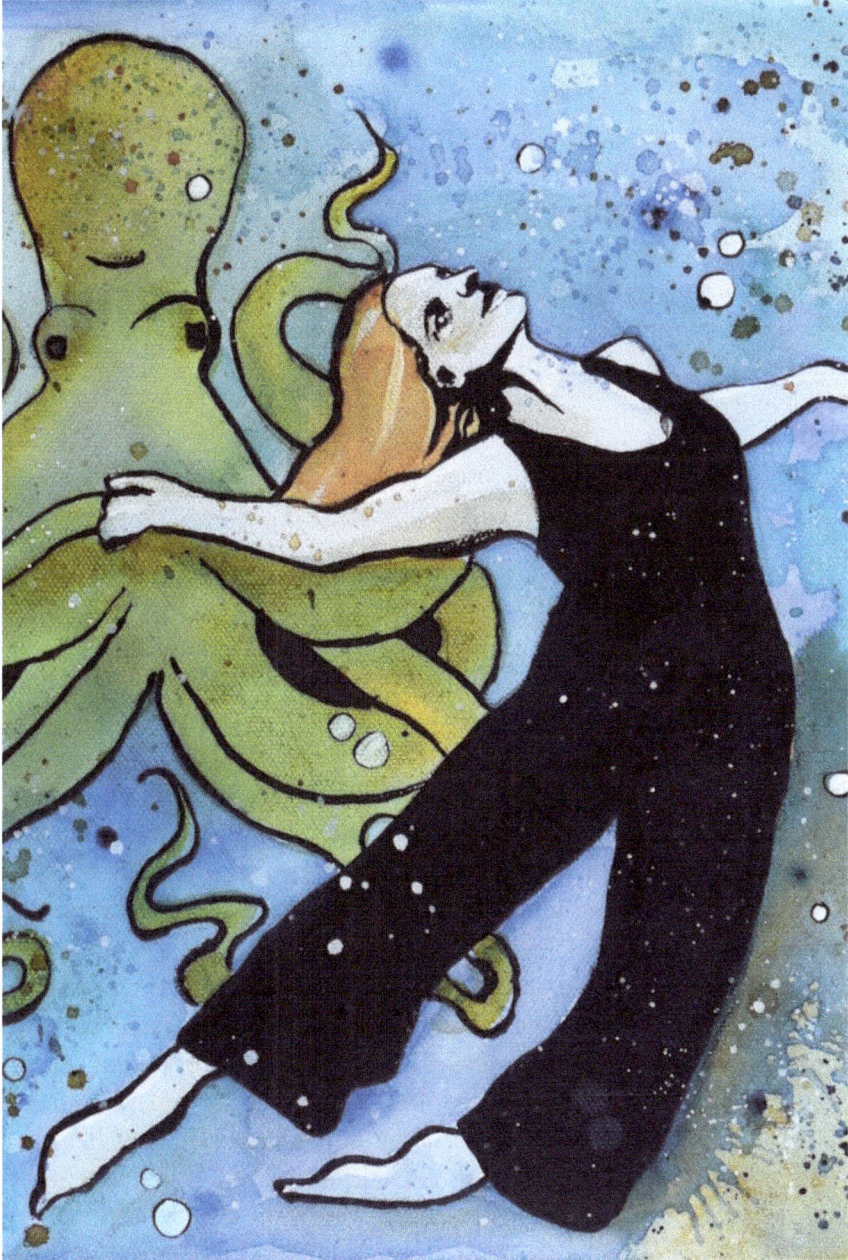

## Tend Your Altar

The season of Ostara, also known as the vernal equinox, marks the first day of spring and the halfway point between the solstices. For those of us in the northern hemisphere, Ostara falls between March 19th and 22nd. This ancient holiday honors resurrection, renewal, and fresh, warm energy as the sun crosses the celestial equator, moving from south to north. I don't want to make any of the other holidays feel bad, but I have to admit that the equinoxes are my favorite on the wheel of the year.

Winter is over. Spring has sprung. And it's time to rearrange our seasonal altar in honor of the vernal equinox. This is an opportunity to capture the verdant and expectant nature of the season and ritualize our creative emergence. But first, let's get out into the great wide open and see what Mother Nature has on offer.

This year for the Vernal Equinox, I was up in time to witness the sunrise. My Celtic ancestors did this for thousands of years in celebration of the vernal equinox. I drove into the mountains to escape a thick fog that settled overnight on the valley floor. I parked at the summit that bridges Pine and Eagle Valleys to watch the sun crest. It first appeared as a pink and wheat-colored lateral flash illuminating the distance over the Seven Devils of Western Idaho. Then it really opened up — a white sheet of light blurring the vista before me. I inhaled the cool air and felt the muscles between my scapula release.

The ancient Celts worshiped solar holidays on hills crowned with standing stones. I don't have a stone circle handy, so I made my way to Eagle Creek, a place that boasts a congregation of boulders. Eagle Creek is fed by the glacial melt of the Wallowa Mountains and its clarity at this time of year gives it the appearance of beveled glass. Large stones, sometimes twenty feet tall, have settled at the creek's edge.

I squatted down with one hand on a boulder to steady myself as I reached through the glinting water to pull out small blue-gray river rocks. I skipped the flat ones across the water and I slid the round ones into my coat pocket to take home for my altar. These water-worn stones have spent years and years tumbled by seasonal creek flow. Their once rough edges have been smoothed and polished over time. They have endured ice, fire, wind, and water. The storms and turmoil they've weathered make them all the more beautiful. Just like us, I suppose.

Ostara is a Teutonic Earth goddess of Germanic origin who was adopted by the Anglo-Saxons. And it is her name that marks the vernal equinox. But I want to honor the story of another goddess — not Ostara because she gets all the attention at this time of year — but a lesser known Irish witch called Cailleach Buí. *Cailleach* is Gaelic for hag or witch and she is one of the oldest figures in Celtic mythology. She holds within her the wisdom of the ages. There are several figures that bear strong similarities to the Cailleach found in other European cultures, especially in Germanic and Slavic traditions such as Frau Holle and Baba Yaga.

In Loughcrew, Ireland, there is a sacred cairn, which is a kind of hilled tomb, known as *Sliabh na Calliagh* (the Mountain of the Witch). At dawn on the Spring Equinox, a sunbeam enters the chamber of the cairn and strikes a stone, which bears ancient carvings that are thought to be a kind of star map or astral guide. The carvings date back to 3500 and 3300 BC.

The legend says that the Cailleach Buí, had an apron full of stones, and as she leapt from hill to hill, she scattered the stones and boulders across the land, creating the great cairns of Ireland. Many believe that she is buried beneath the stone cairn at Loughcrew.

It is the Cailleach Buí I think of now as I hop from stone to stone along Eagle Creek. With stones in my pocket and ancient waters running past my feet, I am mirroring the actions of my ancestors, inviting their wisdom to flow through me. It is the morning of the vernal equinox and halfway across the world in Loughcrew, a beam of light has pierced the dark cave of the Cailleach's cairn. And here I am, with my body resting, creekside near an ancient boulder, connected to an ancestral line that runs back through the ages.

## ALTAR PRACTICE

Let's prepare our altar to greet the muse of spring. Some Celtic people call her Kore, pregnant with possibility, and others look to Brigid, the creative midwife. If I were to prepare for a birthing mother, I'd play some soft music and dim the lights. I'd warm the water for tea, stock the ice for drinks and cold compresses, and lay down protective sheeting on the bed for when delivery was imminent. What might we need to prepare for the arrival of the muse? Perhaps a favorite ink pen? A clean desk? A fresh set of knitting needles? A new pair of gardening gloves? I like to go through all of my acrylic paints and pick the dried paint off the lids and give each one a good shake. This lets them know that it's almost go-time. Sometimes I even make a playlist of musical selections to welcome the muse and celebrate her arrival.

When your room preparations feel complete, make your way to your seasonal altar. Take stock of the objects. Some items will remain and be rearranged. Others will be removed and stored for next year. Take a moment to lovingly dust or wipe down the surface and remaining objects with a cloth. And as you do this, hold this question close to your heart: *How does inner wisdom flow through me?*

Sit for a moment at your altar. Let the air fall in and out of your body without force. What does the muse of spring crave as an offering on the altar? Creek water? River rocks? A bloom? An egg? Perhaps your altar will evolve over the course of the next six weeks, with new flowers each week as they bloom forth in your part of the world.

Once you've arranged your objects, light a candle and find a comfortable place beside your altar to sit or stand. Gaze upon the objects. Where are your people from? What waters, rivers, streams, or wells did they worship at? Where are their sacred hills? Which goddesses birthed their landscapes? Which wise woman revealed their truths?

Let this vernal equinox be an invitation to reach back through your lineage, chosen or by birth, and pick up the stones left by your ancestors along your path. You are the dream they conjured at the water's edge and they are the earthen shoulders on which you stand. You are a conduit through which their wisdom flows. And the creative process you are nurturing is a pathway for that inner wisdom to spring forth.

SKETCHBOOK PRACTICE

The poet Mary Oliver tells us that to pay attention is our endless and proper work. But what does "paying attention" mean? This will be different for each one of us. For me it means an active journal practice. This is why we set out on *The Creative Alchemy Cycle* path in Imbolc with the journal as a way to record our deep noticing. The journal is a way to nurture a continual creative practice, no matter what you're making, writing, weaving, and growing.

This season we'll expand our journal practice to include a sketchbook. (They can be one in the same!) A sketchbook is a place where we can explore and expand the boundaries of what we see and how we see it. For me, it's how I understand my own preferences: what I love, what I look at, what I notice, what I obsess over. My grandmother Orma Minshull was a watercolorist and she always told me "Draw what you notice and notice what you draw." She taught me that this was the process by which artists develop and hone their artistic taste and personal style.

So let's take inventory of everything we see during the season of Ostara: feathers, twigs, leaves, river rocks, green shoots, husks, threadbare leaves from last winter's mulch, cloud formations, bud-like nodules on twigs, and the like. Let's capture these items in the form of quick drawings or sketches. This is a wonderful way to get to know these objects and become comfortable replicating their shape, color, and personality. A sketchbook is a place to play and explore. These are not finished pieces and do not carry the weight of "completed work" or "art." Your sketchbook is a creative laboratory for creating your own visual and imagistic vocabulary. It's a way to absorb the energy of all you see and better understand your relationship with them.

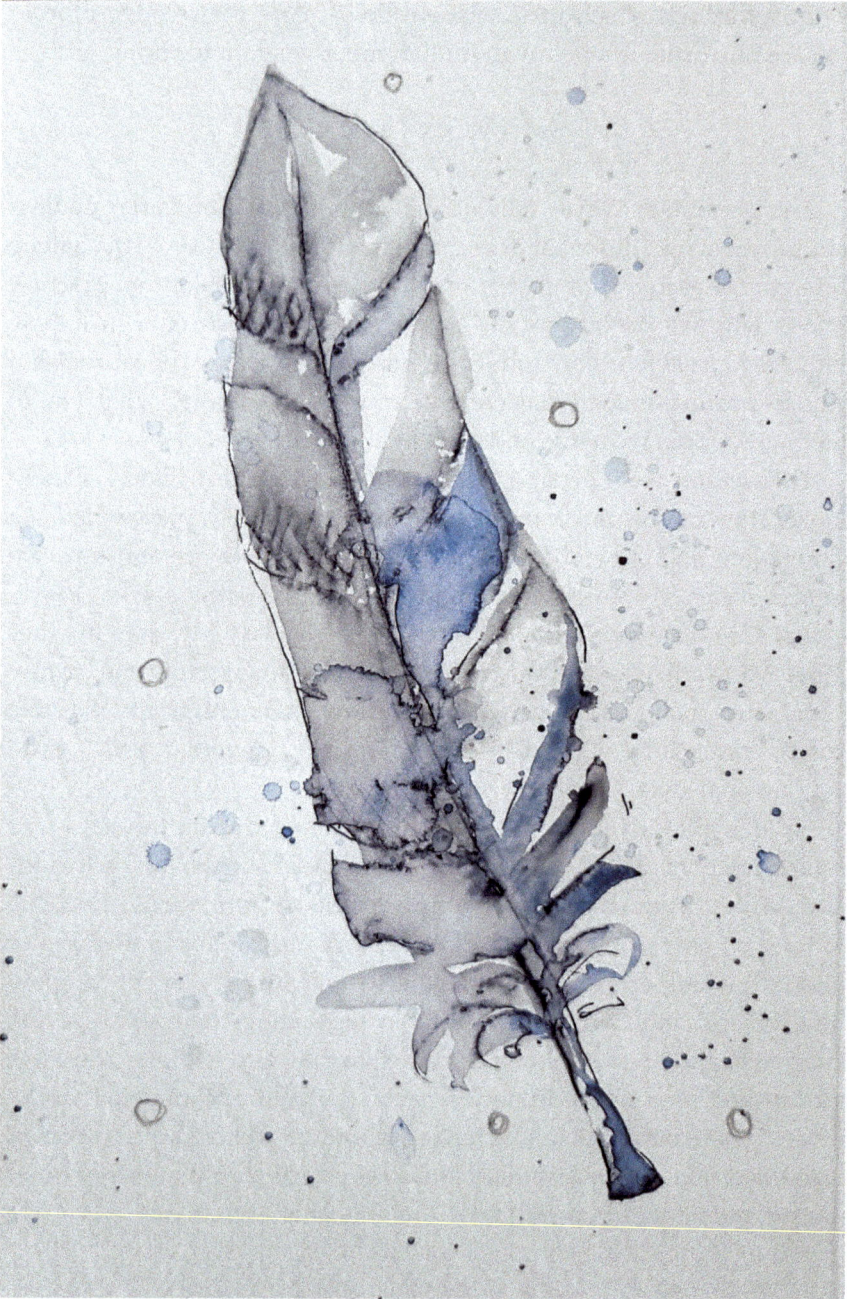

## Incubation

When I need extra holding and healing, or the world is caving in a bit, I always turn to my sketchbook. My sketchbook practice is a powerful tool for slowing down and rendering my thoughts visible.

This season I'm exploring feathers. The molting eagles and kestrels of Imboc have dropped some beauties. Feathers hold deep significance for me. My brother, who died in 2014, liked to create 3D artworks with feathers. In memory, I had a feather tattooed on my inner forearm, tied around my wrist with a string that bears his name. He's always there, holding my hand, close to my pulse, reminding me to fly.

If you are new to sketchbook practice, breathe into the excitement of being a beginner and remember that it's all about process. And if you are already a keeper of doodles and drawings, then allow your practice to deepen your relationship with the physical world around you. Let's begin with a water ritual to ground us in the powerful now.

The cardiovascular system of any landscape is its waterways. Just like in the human body, creeks, rivers, lakes, and wells are a kind of lifeblood, delivering oxygen and energy into its deepest corners. Water is not only our life source, but also our teacher. I come from people who made annual pilgrimages to holy wells where they sang prayer songs into the water and drank deep its blessings. For my ancestors, breath and song reverberating in a holy well was a magical combination that allowed the prayer to travel through the consciousness of Earth in the form of water.

All water is connected to all water. Not only does it travel through space in the form of groundwater, rivers, and oceans, but it also travels through time because it's always been the same water. Sure we may have picked up some water along the way, but we live in a closed system. All of the water that was ever here on Earth is connected molecularly to all water everywhere. If you pour yourself a glass of water, you can know that all of your ancestors have imbibed that same water. It goes beyond interconnectedness and expands to what Tibetan Buddhist teacher Thich Naht Hanh calls interbeing. Not that we are simply connected to water / tree / stone, but that we are water / tree / stone.

Pour yourself a glass of water and take it in hand. You can close your eyes if you wish or simply soften your gaze. Let air drop into your body and fill you up. Then let it naturally drop out, noticing the wave of air that comes in, and the wave of air that flows out.

Gratitude for the Earth that cradles us.
Gratitude for the Breath that connects us.
Gratitude for the Fire in our hearts that bind us.
Gratitude for the Water in our hands that fuels us.

Take a moment to hold your own unique gratitudes in mind. Make sure that you are named among your gratitudes. Speak them aloud. Let them travel into the water you hold, knowing that this is the same water held by others in your circle, others in your community, and others in your long and unceasing lineage. Softly flutter your eyes open. Drink deep this life-giving gift, filled with gratitude, and the goodness of this moment. Enjoy the sensation of water in your mouth, the coolness, the fluidity, the pure magic of its existence. Repeat this ritual as often as you like.

## Action

I live in a place called Pine Valley in a house called Pine Cottage. Before moving to Eastern Oregon, I never lived among conifers. Now, they are an enormous part of my everyday life. Every single window in my home gives way to a Ponderosa, Douglas or Norway fir. We are, in essence, surrounded.

Conifers are some of the oldest forms of plant life on earth. Researchers found traces of conifers dated back to 300 million years ago. They've taught me that we are short and the world is long. Pine trees and pine cones have since made their way into many of my sketches and therefore many of my paintings. Some folks who know my work well even associate my work now with conifers. This is absolutely a product of where I live and what objects fill my eyeballs and sketchbook.

**Which natural objects or botanicals surround you? Are there any natural objects or botanicals you seem to notice more than others?**

Once, during a particularly windy March, a 90-foot Ponderosa uprooted along our soggy fence line and fell onto our house. (Thank you, old man Thompson.) I absolutely love the trees that surround my home, but this was a shock and our home was badly damaged. To ease my worry and alchemize my anxiety into something more manageable, I painted an "I still love you" watercolor of the remaining pine trees into my sketchbook. It was an act of reclaiming my own sense of safety and honoring the trees that were still on their feet after the storm. A "thank you for protecting us" painting. An "I forgive you, I know you didn't mean it, and I understand why you did it" painting.

Sketching the Ponderosa allowed me to enter into a kind of conversation with the tree – a tree that literally came into our home, demanding that I pay attention to its story, its history, its needs, and its legacy. I began to experience our creative intimacy, however complicated, as a pathway for its wisdom to flow through me.

**Have you ever lost a tree or a garden or a harvest? Perhaps painting a portrait or writing a letter to this fallen friend might help ease the hurt.**

In addition to painting an homage to the fallen Ponderosa, I became obsessed with sharing its seeds, the pine cone, with friends. In the months that followed I used pine cones as paper weights, decorations, window jambs, and I even used the smaller Douglas fir pine cones in place of Styrofoam peanuts when shipping packages. I wanted to reclaim my relationship with these trees, nourish our connection, and better understand them by drawing them closer.

**Pick a botanical element that is meaningful to you. It could be laven-**

der, hay, daphne, leaves, or cedar. Robin Wall Kimmerer chose Sweet-grass to begin her most famous book. Hold it up to your nose. Can you smell it? Breathe it in. What do you feel when you look at this object? What other images come to you? Set it near you if you can. Or if it's not something you can hold (say, a Ponderosa), set yourself near enough that you can take it in with your senses. If you want to stay in your journal, then free-write about your experience of this object or element. And if you're exploring your sketchbook, begin drawing. If sketching makes you feel a bit wobbly, then proceed to the next prompt and we'll create a little scaffolding around your first sketch.

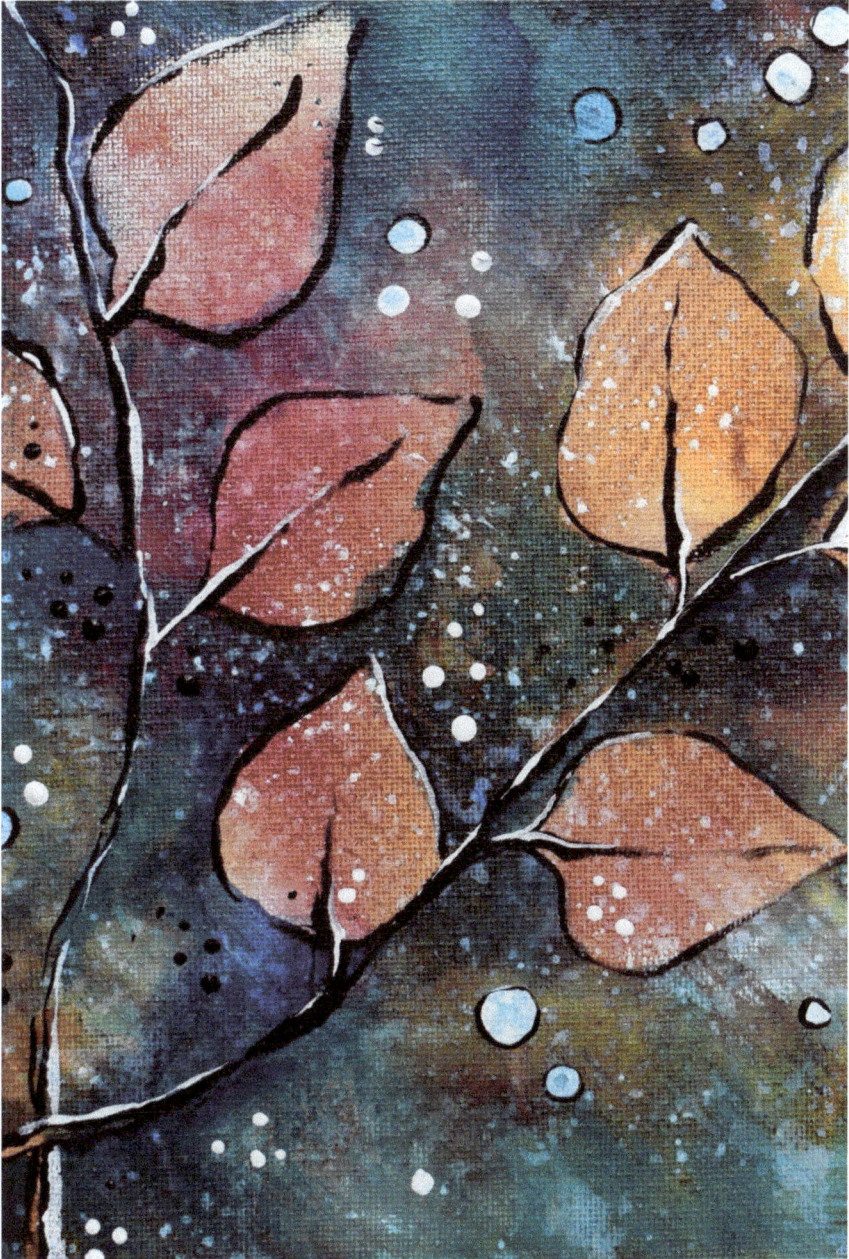

Most children, when asked to draw something representational like a house or a tree, begin with a line. It's a quick and intuitive way to create form, define edges, build structure, and lead the eye from one part of an object to another. As we begin to build our own visual vocabulary and capture the essence of objects we are in relationship with, line drawing is an excellent place to start.

## Line Drawing

The key to line drawing is to allow your hand to lay down the line that you actually see. If someone asked me to draw an eye without looking at an actual eye, it would look very simple: a pupil, an iris, and the curved upper and lower edge of the eyelid. Voilà, an eye! And you would recognize it as an eye, albeit somewhat cartoonish. But the practice I'm asking us to participate in is one of deep noticing. Really look at your object and sketch what is physically there. This means that you'll look more at your object than you will at your drawing. When I am intentional about noticing the object in front of me, my line drawing is slow. I start small and work my way out.

I might begin with the iris. I notice the starburst pattern around the pupil and the irregularity at the edge of the circle of the pupil (a sign of astigmatism). My hand follows what I see. Part of the white of the eye is shrouded with heavy lashes, and I draw accordingly. I make my way along the bottom lid noticing that there is an inner line where the ball meets the skin and an outer line where the lash line begins. My hand follows suit. And then the soft swooping handle of the tear duct. Were a child to see my drawing, they might ask if the tear duct is the state of Florida hanging off of my overly-round map of the United States. But no matter. I am practicing intentional seeing.

## Blind Contour

Want to try something wonderfully fun and illuminating? A blind contour drawing is made up of lines that are drawn without ever looking at your paper. This forces you to study your subject closely, observing every shape and edge with your eyes, as your hand mimics these on paper. The aim is not to produce a realistic image (is it ever?), but rather to strengthen the connection between eyes, hand and brain. Blind contour is a very effective way to strengthen our capacity to truly see.

## Gesture Drawing

For those of us interested in capturing an object in motion like a bird or child, try gesture drawing. A gesture drawing is completed quickly – often in short timed durations, such as 20, 30, 60 or 90 seconds – using fast, expressive lines. Gesture drawings capture basic forms and proportions. It's a great way to capture the essence of a subject without focusing on detail. This type of drawing helped me to increase my drawing speed, confidence and intuitive mark-making skill.

As you know, I'm an avid journaler. I make it a point to sit down every day and put pen to paper. But sometimes, I just don't feel like writing. And some days my analytical mind gets in the way of my natural creative flow. That's when I turn to other techniques that help me step away from linear thinking and engage the associative part of my brain. Two of my favorite journaling practices are clustering and collage, because they always help me to reclaim the natural joy that comes from drawing connections between what I see, feel, and think. This ultimately sharpens my taste and style and reveals my subterranean creative cravings.

## Clustering

How do ideas correlate? Which creative impulses connect to others? These are questions I frequently have about my own creative process. Clustering is a technique developed by Gabriele Lusser Rico and shared in her book *Writing the Natural Way*. Clustering (or mapping as it is sometimes called) can help you become aware of different ways to think about a subject. It's a stream-of-consciousness exercise that acts as a doorway to your ideas. It has also been very useful to me when my writing or painting process feels blocked.

To create a cluster, write a word in the center of your paper. It could be a name, a feeling, or a memory, or any other subject you'd like to explore. Circle it. Then, using the whole sheet of paper, rapidly jot down other ideas and associations related to your central word or image. If an idea spawns other ideas, link them together using lines and circles to form a cluster of ideas. The whole purpose here is to use lines and circles to show visually how your ideas relate to one another and to your main subject. This process should take no more than a couple of minutes. I like to use this as a prewriting tool, but I have also used it in my sketchbook for creating related imagery. It is a fast and effective way to knit together disparate ideas. I find that this technique also helps to strengthen my associative thinking and expand my creative options. Give it a try!

## Collage

While line drawing is a wonderful way to capture the essence of an object in real time, collage can sometimes be better suited for creating imagery around a feeling, emotion, or sense. The thing I love about collage is I don't need to come up with my own words and imagery. I have full permission to use the words and images created by others. Instead of being the source material, I get to step into the role of curator.

**Collect Your Materials:** All you'll need for collage work is a pair of scissors, a glue stick, your sketchbook, and paper ephemera from which to curate your image. I have a file in my office filled with clippings, decorative papers, magazine images, and other bits of paper. Sometimes I also hang onto theater tickets, interesting clothing tags, and other random bits. Whenever I see something that pleases my eye or captures my imagination, I cut it out and slip it into the file. I never ask why I like it, I just heed the impulse and tuck it away for later.

**Select Your Images:** If you don't have a file of pre-curated materials, then feel free to comb through some magazines and cut out images that appeal to you. This intuitive selection process usually takes me about thirty minutes. When you see an image or words that speak to you for any reason, cut it out and set it aside. Think of it as spirit speaking to you through the available images you've got at your fingertips. Do not judge what you love or what you are drawn to. Simply notice your connection to it and cut it out. You may or may not end up using it in your collage, but cut it out anyway. This is about creating a visual vocabulary on which to build your collage.

**Arrange Your Images:** I usually separate my images into three piles. One for pictures of objects (people, plants, animals). One for backgrounds (textures, patterns). And another for text, words, and letters. I like to begin by pouring over my images and selecting ones that are particularly evocative. As you pull these images together, you'll notice that they begin to tell their own kind of story. I also like to keep a guiding word or phrase in mind when I'm arranging a collage, especially if I'm creating a collage to reflect a feeling, emotion, or state of being.

Take time to play with where you want each piece of paper to go. Arrange and rearrange. Where do things overlap? Where are they superimposed? How are you layering color? Texture? Refrain from gluing anything down until you have a strong sense of what needs to be glued down first. Collage is a process of building from the ground up. Base layers tend to be made up of your texture and pattern pile. Middle layers tend to be made up of objects and images of people, animals, plants, or places. And the final layer tends to be words. And of course, rules were meant to be broken. Allow this to be an intuitive process. The painter Flora Bowley likes to ask her students, "What are you craving next?" This is a great question to keep in your mind's eye as you collage. What color am I craving next? What shape? What word? What feeling?

And as always, feel free to write your own words. If your collage, sketch, or line drawing illuminates an idea for you, grab your pen and journal about it. Your sketchbook and journal are interchangeable.

### INTEGRATION

The drawing and sketchbook techniques I describe above might be new for you. So before we continue, I want to address a feeling that may be coming up. When I am learning something new or stretching my skill set in unpracticed ways, I frequently bump up against my own limiting beliefs. For me, a limiting belief is usually a negative or self-critical thought I have about myself, that not only weakens my sense of self-worth but holds me back from a feeling of belonging. Belonging isn't something you can buy or receive from someone else. Belonging is a bone-deep knowing that you are right where you're supposed to be. Limiting beliefs sabotage my creative work and "other" me from my own inner knowing. They keep me from living into the fullness of my life and prevent me from doing, being, and saying the things I long to do, be, and say.

As we deepen our sketchbook practice and make friends with the unknown, let's spend some time journaling about how our limiting beliefs trip us up. And more importantly, let's explore how we might counteract them. The truth is that limiting beliefs are a kind of noise, created by external oppressive systems and cycles, meant to distract us from claiming our power. Here are some questions that have come up for me, that might be useful as we continue to expand our creative practice:

**What stories have you been telling yourself about what you can and cannot do?**

**What stories have you been telling yourself about what others can and cannot do?**

**How do those stories protect you from being hurt?**

**Who would you be and what would you do if these beliefs were not true? (Pssst, they're not true.)**

I am a person who spends a lot of time in my head. (Oh, you too?) This is a great place for inception and inspiration. But it is an ineffective place for doing the damn thing. There is no substitute for the action we seek. We cannot learn to swim if we are not in the water. And we cannot expand our capacity to write if we are not in the notebook. And we cannot develop our visual vocabulary if we're not at the canvas. That's why a robust journal and sketchbook practice is key for our creative work in the world. These practices provide a resilient space to experiment and translate thought into action. It will also be a place for us to track our own transformation and notice patterns of growth, grief, and gratitude.

I want to expand the journal questions I offered above. Let's show our limiting beliefs the door and engage in some creative alchemy:

**Choose one limiting belief – the ickiest story you keep telling yourself – that you don't want to carry with you into the future. Pick something that is shielding your light from the world. Write this limiting belief a goodbye letter. I like to think of it as a break up letter. Start your letter with a salutation and go from there.**

### One-Word Prompts for Ostara

Wave • Shapeshift • Resurrection • Water • Witness
Sketch • Sunrise • Ritual • Selkie • Process
Spring • Dive • Flow • Alchemy • Tide
Undertow • Crave • Collage • Prayer • Salt
Float • Stone • Vernal • Green • Celestial
Myth • Creek • Crone • Fecundity • Sacred

### The Next Six Weeks

Spring makes me sentimental. D.H. Lawrence once referred to sentimentality as giving something more tenderness than God would. But if I were to guess, I bet God has a tender spot in her heart for spring and its many gifts. During the weeks ahead, let your sentimentality lead the way. Carry your sketchbook (or a camera) wherever you go. Capture the fleeting moment, the greening of Earth, the swelling bud, the beetle, the brash buzzing of life. Sketch its essence onto a page in the book of your heart. Collage and carve a pathway for its wisdom to flow forth.

The time between the spring equinox and Beltane is roughly six weeks. Find an unfurling flower. Watch it grow. Draw it down.

Perhaps you sketch or photograph it every day. Or watch the waves and chart the tides. Or perhaps you'll map the rising sun and sketch down the moment it appears over your neighbor's roof top, shifting slightly north each morning. Whatever you choose, become its student. Apprentice yourself to the wisdom it offers. Wade into its waters, become susceptible to its pull, and let it tumble you like a stone.

## CROSS THE THRESHOLD

As I write this, there is a full moon in the sky. It's often called the Worm Moon, because this is the time of year when the soil comes alive again with microbial movement. The worms of the Earth are busy transforming yesterday's decay into tomorrow's growth. This full moon calls me to re-tune my ear to the living earth. It calls me, despite my limiting beliefs, to face my time squarely in the eye, to notice the rot as well as the renewal, the collapse as well as the co-arising.

This is the season of resurrection. Everything is coming alive. And just like the Cailleach's cairn at Loughcrew, the opening of the cave of my heart has aligned with the sun and everything is suddenly illuminated. It's vulnerable work, shedding light in dark corners. We risk being truly seen. When we stretch ourselves, try new things, and follow pathways we've never explored, it's natural to feel exposed and wobbly. When you feel unsteady, let your natural curiosity lead the way. Follow your creative cravings.

Follow the sound of a creek.
Follow the curve of a stone.
Follow the spine of a feather.
Follow the vein of a leaf.
Follow the arch of the sun.
Follow the rise of a wave.
Follow.
Follow.
Follow.

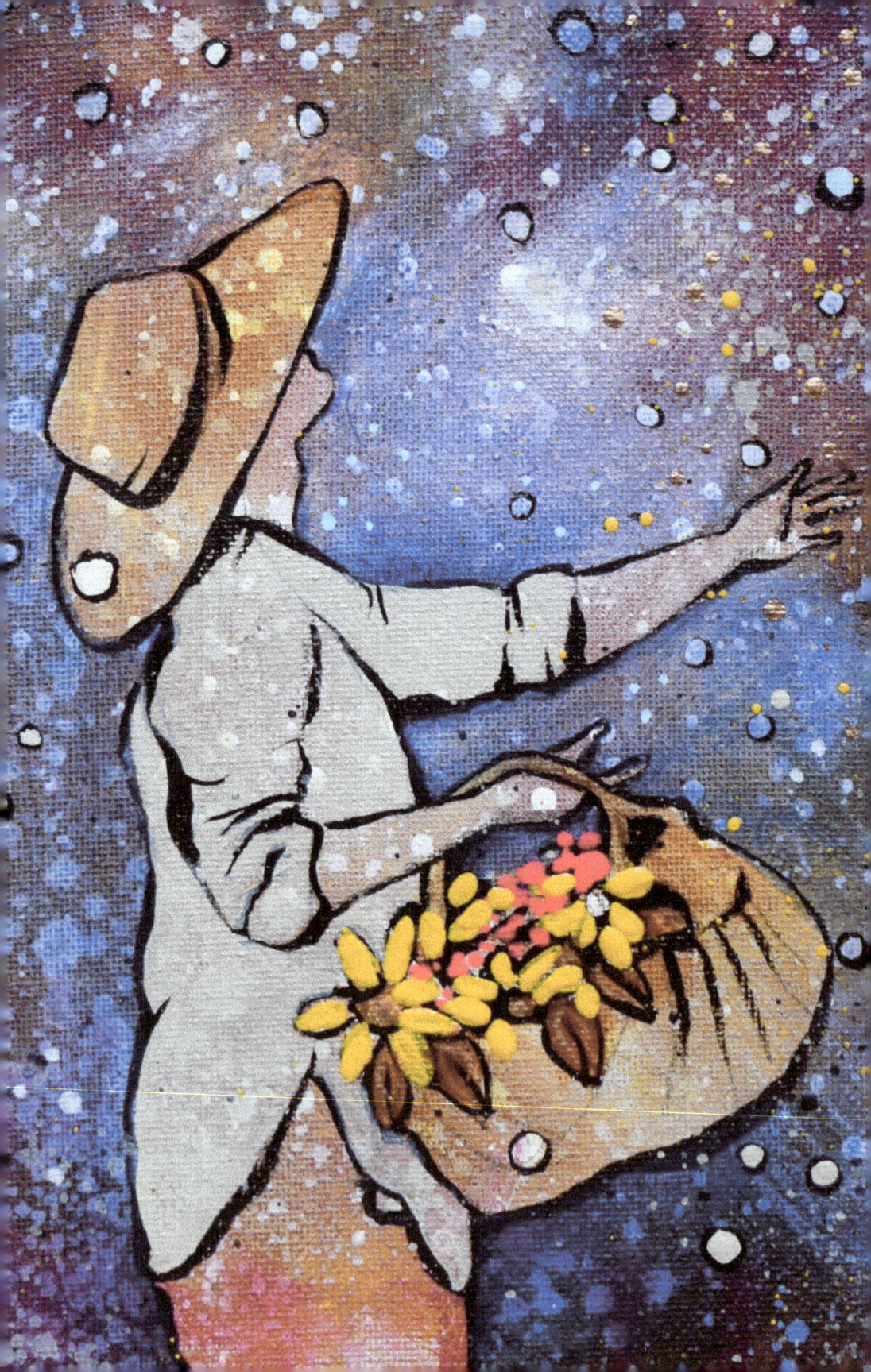

4

# WE ARE FLOWERS: BELTANE

## EMBODIMENT PRACTICE

**The Call:** Home is in your body.

**The Question:** How can I cultivate belonging?

**The Time:** May 1st

**The Origin:** Beltane is an ancient fire festival, often called May Day, that marks the midway point between the vernal equinox and the summer solstice.

**The Imagery:** Flower, Blossom, Garden, Sun

**The Themes:** Creative Cross-Pollination, Pleasure, Embodiment, and Belonging

DO YOU HEAR THE CALL? ALL LIFE IS BURSTING FORTH NOW. NO LONGER the timid shoots of early spring, searching, desperate for light, pressing through Earth's cold crust, but the hot and bothered expansion of leafy canopies, heavy-lidded flowers, opening their saturated inner folds to any pollinator that happens by. The world is ripe and anticipatory. If you can hear over the wild patter of Earth's heartbeat, there is a hum – a low tone in sync with the harmonic buzzing of the bees, mayflies, and wasps. This is the thrum of life. It is the blood pumping through your veins. Your body is not separate from this Earth. Your body is a creative conduit, a threshold through which you may perceive the world. It was built for sensation, a gift given to you by Mother Earth herself.

The next six weeks are an invitation to pause and ritualize the art of noticing. We'll explore a variety of invitations for the body to unfurl and disclose its wisdom. Beltane gives us permission to seek a sacred kind of embodied joy through the portal of our senses. Let's crown ourselves with flowers, sneak away to the tent with our lovers, commit to our own blossoming, step into the fire, and embrace the pleasures of the season.

CALLING YOU HOME – A SEASONAL HOMILY FOR BELTANE

Many years ago, I was invited to a May Day wedding for a dear high school friend. Callie was a lanky, blond, waifish creature who excelled at math, science, and swimming. Her hair was always green in the summer. I often thought that she might really be a mermaid. She was marrying Gabriel, her high school sweetheart, a beachy beauty who spent his formative years surfing in the Pacific and hiking the coastal mountain ranges above San Luis Obispo. His hands were always calloused from weekend landscaping he did alongside his father. He smelled of seaweed, salt, and marijuana.

Callie's family had a beautiful piece of unincorporated land tucked away near Nacimiento Lake in Central California. *Nacimiento* is Spanish for birth. Perfect for a May Day wedding. After turning off the highway, I followed the dirt road into an arid landscape dotted with live oak, sage, and juniper. Ground squirrels popped in and out of sight. Gold and rust-red ribbons were tied to crooked fence posts and tree trunks, inviting me further and further away from the main road and towards the nuptial site. The road ended in a long u-shaped clearing and I parked my car along with the others. I swung my legs around the driver's seat, set my feet on the bare earth, and walked towards the music.

I came to a gathering of Black Oak trees that looked like they'd circled up just for the wedding. Their limbs stretched out across the expanse and created a dappled canopy. The space was pulsing with djembe drumming, women grooving to the reggae style rhythm in long skirts, and men standing around an open fire pit. The flames leapt above their heads and the slow rippling waves of heat created a wonderful visual distortion of the trees beyond. As I took in the scene I could see all of the elements of Beltane on display: ochre, crimson and cream colored flowers stuffed into earthen bowls, a large central bonfire, feast food, dancing, music, and a make-shift bar in the back of a truck serving honey mead.

The drumming kicked up a notch, alerting those gathered to a transition. Callie and Gabriel appeared at the edge of the circle, adorned with ribbons and floral crowns. A host of women in yellow dresses led the bride and groom - the maiden and her bridegroom - through the crowd while children spread blossoms out before them. I felt in that moment the ancient presence of the May Queen, goddess of fertility.

Beltane is the spring counterpart to Samhain. While in the autumn everything is dying, in spring it comes alive. It is during this ancient holiday when the May Queen weds the King of the Forest. The term "Beltane" is derived from the Celtic god named Bel and the Gaelic word "teine" which means fire. Together, Beltane means "Bright Fire". Is there anything brighter or more stuffed with possibility than a public declaration of love? Beltane reminds us that ceremonies need not be solemn to be sacred. There is deep divinity and power in an act of collective mirth.

I joined the wedding guests and we followed the couple. We were led to the far edge of the clearing where the father of the groom had constructed a wooden arbor with an image of the rising sun carved into the arch. The couple reached the flower strewn altar and stood under the rising sun. They kissed long and hard and turned to face us. I remember thinking, "A wedding that *starts* with a kiss is my kind of wedding!" It all felt so celebratory and permissive.

Callie and Gabriel spoke aloud their commitment to grow together, play together, to raise a family together, and to accept the love and cherished wisdom of their community. They kissed again as we showered them with petals and shouts of adoration.

I thought the ceremony was coming to an end, when Callie stepped down from the altar. She addressed the guests, "We're ready to start a family!" We cheered. I had never seen such a forward and centered bride. Her lips were swollen from kissing and the white petals of the wreath encircling her head gleamed in the late afternoon sun.

Then the most incredible thing happened. We followed the bride of spring and her beautiful groom from the altar to a white canvas tent tucked under the oaks beyond the bonfire. There was a hand painted sign above the threshold into the tent that read, "We belong to each other." And at that moment, I knew it was true. It was true not only of the bride and groom, but of those gathered. And it was true for the Black Oaks that enshrouded the tent, and the warblers tucked away in their own love-nests, and the ground squirrels hiding from our thunderous noise, and the newts in the nearby creek, and the dragonfly larvae bobbing in the eddy, and the mistletoe hanging in the overstory, and everything. We belong to each other.

Wildflower seed packets were passed around from guest to guest and we were encouraged to toss the seeds onto the tent as a blessing for their union. The couple ducked their heads into the tent and the guests headed back to the fire. It had never occurred to me to publicly ritualize the first time a couple made love as husband and wife. What a revelation!

As I stood gazing at the tent that sheltered their love, I felt a pang of regret ripple through my chest. When in my life had I ever been so free and open with my own feelings? When had I ever felt such permission to reveal my need for love and belonging? When had I ever been allowed to indulge my senses, enjoy my own vitality, or make choices in such an embodied way? In my world, especially as a young woman, my physical prowess and sexuality was not for sharing. And because I was encouraged to hide these essential parts of my being, I was fearful and ashamed of true surrender. But here were two souls, embodying the divine mother and her consort, tapping into an ancient May Day tradition. The reality of their union and the myth they invoked revealed to me the essential power of ritual as a means for transformation. I was gob-smacked.

While the couple made love, the guests relished other pleasures. We feasted. We laughed. We sang a toast to the couple, danced, and welcomed them back into community after their time in the tent. Callie and Gabriel gave themselves to each other, and in doing so, they gave us all permission to love deeper, share bigger, and surrender to our truest nature.

This Beltane, welcome the May Queen and her consort into your home, into your bedroom, and into your heart. Where are the places in your life where you can say yes with your whole body? Trust your aliveness. Pay attention to what you crave. Bloom forth. Leave the shadows of winter behind and step into the center of your belonging.

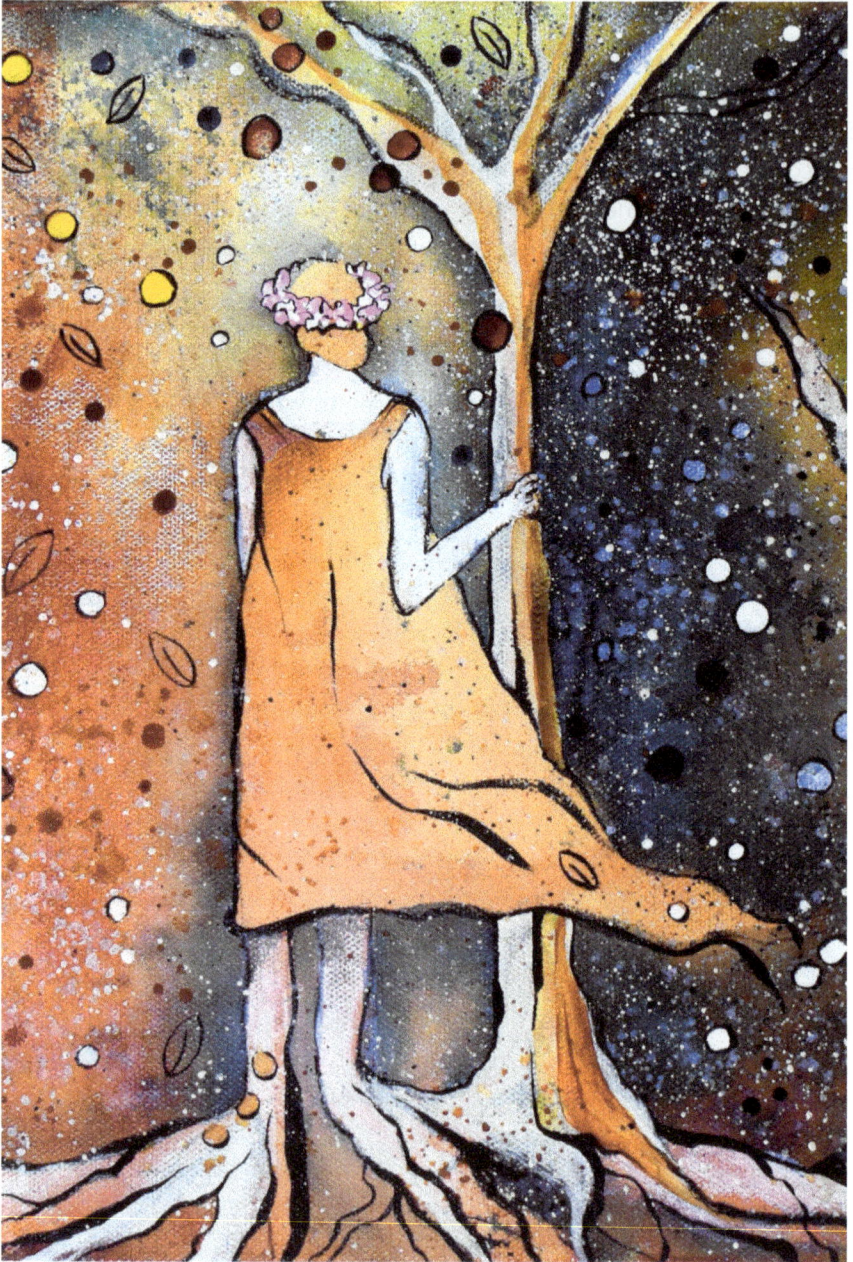

## Tend the Altar

Beltane marks the midway point between the vernal equinox and the summer solstice. This ancient holiday honors passion, flowering, love, color, and all things sensual. My Grandma Jane always called it "sexy season". And it's true. Everything and everyone seems a little randy in May.

This season, I invite you to consider your body as altar. How might you enter a room or prepare a meal or choose clothing or talk to yourself if you knew that your body was holy ground? To honor the body as altar, we must first treat it as sacred and then apprentice ourselves to its wisdom. And its wisdom can only be known through the senses.

The senses are our greatest allies when it comes to our creativity. If we spiral back in our lineage, we find that our ancestors had sharp senses, used as a means of survival as well as creative adaptation. In her book *Merchants of Light*, Betty J. Kovács traces the loss of our sensorial prowess to Christian colonizers who persecuted land-based people by squashing indigenous ways of knowing and destroying our ancient customs, ways of dress, languages, and spiritual traditions. We've forgotten the power of our senses. We've been conditioned to distrust the information we receive through the lens of our bodies. But our senses are still here, waiting for us to engage and rebuild this fundamental relationship.

So let's get physical. Get down. Get dirty. Sink in. Ritualize sensation. It may be sexy season, but it's also mud between the toes season. Breeze in your hair season. Honey on the lips season. Shed your skin season. Let's once again become intimate with the texture of our aliveness and recognize our bodies as altars.

## Altar Practice

"Home is in your body." I first heard these words spoken by the singer Nai Palm. These five words are, for me, a revelation. As a queer, tall woman of size, I spent most of my young adult life feeling completely outside myself. Never at home in my own skin. Never welcome to adorn myself with fashion or enjoy the body I have been given to walk this Earth. This simple, yet profound statement asks that I rethink old narratives about my body and replace them with new ones. Here are some nurturing ways to reframe old narratives and reclaim our bodies as home:

## Bathe

Wherever I change my seasonal altar, I wipe down the surface with moon water, wash and iron the altar cloth, dust the objects, and burn a little incense. I take my time. I touch it with reverence. I give thanks. Let's do the same with our bodies. Step into the shower or bath. Make it special. Play music or light a candle. Find a wonderful soap or body wash and take a moment with each part of your body. Give thanks aloud for all the work and play each part of you provides. All bodies are good bodies. And all bodies deserve to be loved, touched, cleansed, and honored.

## Adorn

Unless you're a nudist, you get dressed every day. Let's transform this otherwise mundane part of life into a sacred act of expression. My friend Caitlin Quinn practices a kind of magic she calls Wardrobe Resourcery and she says, "Clothing is a necessity, but it can also be an art form. We are evolving at every moment. Our wardrobes can be as fluid as we are." What underclothes, wardrobe items, jewelry, make-up, or hair accessories are calling to you today? What little splash of color do you crave? Intentional adornment is a small but powerful way to remind yourself that you are beloved, deserving of time and attention. You are divine. You have permission to dress the part.

## Nourish

Just as you would lay bread and wine at the feet of a Goddess for prosperity and harvest, fill your plate with offerings of love, bounty, and delicious victuals of praise. Feed your soul. Devour words that weave together the fabric of your wholeness. Savor songs that knit you up and return you to yourself. Imbibe the beauty of the living Earth, a reminder of your own beauty. Feast upon foods that sustain you, nourish you, and delight all your senses. This is no time to count calories. It's time to fill the sanctuary, hydrate the cathedral, and nourish the body as altar. Eat well. Drink deep.

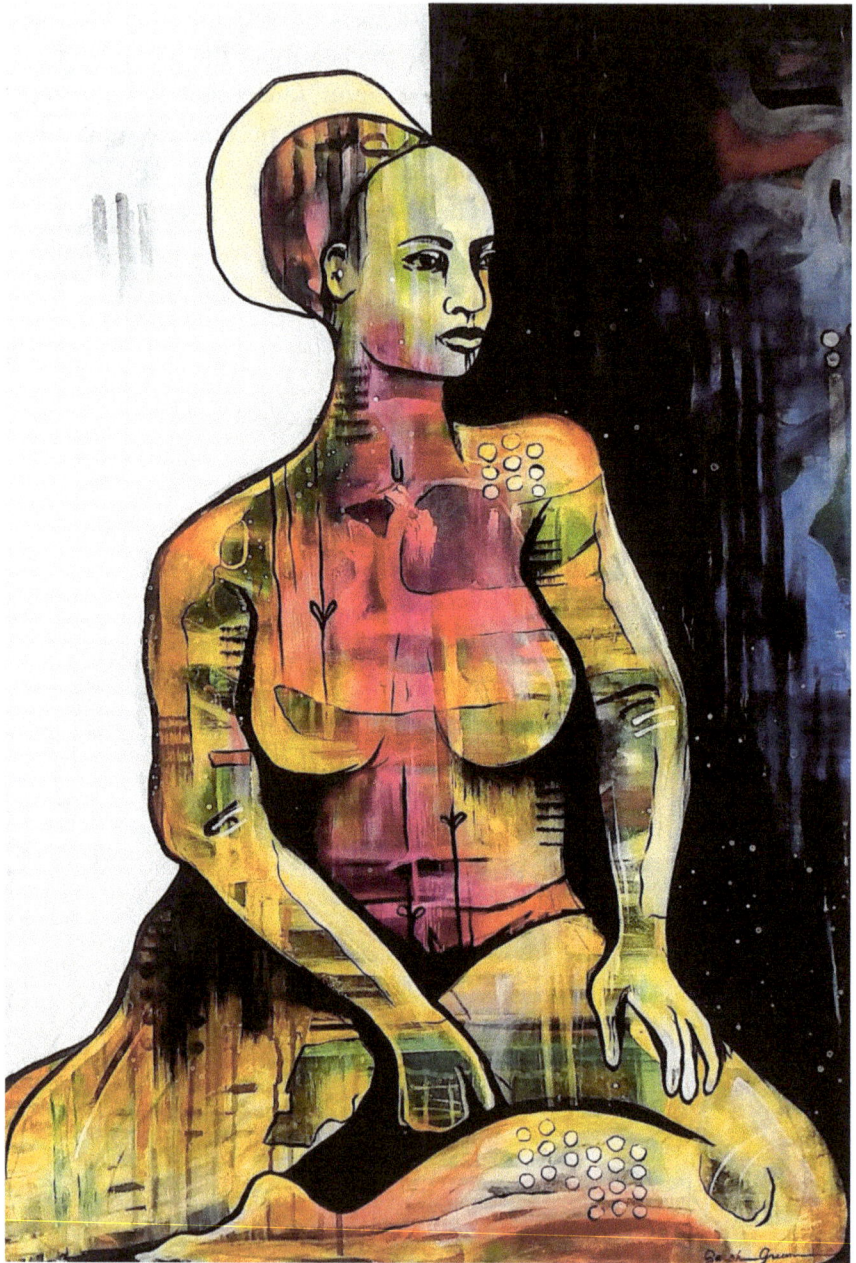

Toni Morrison says it best, "You are your best thing." And you cannot attend to your life's work, your family, your creativity, or your activism in a sustainable way if you are not comfortable in your skin and vibrantly alive. I'm not talking about health, per se, but rather a healthy capacity to feel.

This season *The Creative Alchemy Cycle* is asking us to tap into the deep well of our senses. This means that we must first be on speaking terms with our sensations, able to receive the messages our bodies are sending. During Beltane, sensation is queen. But if our bodies have been shamed or we've been taught to distrust our bodies and ignore physical sensation, then how can we be open to the wisdom our bodies offer?

I'd like to take a moment to also acknowledge that many of us ignore our senses for good reasons. Survivors of abuse and trauma may be consciously or unconsciously gatekeeping their sensorial porosity as a way to protect themselves from further harm. Those of us who are neurodiverse may need to lessen our exposure to overstimulation. You know yourself best. There is no need to "push through" or retraumatize the mind and body. The invitation here is to embrace the alchemical nature of adaptation. We can be both protective and permissive. How can we honor the body as home in ways that feel nourishing, expansive, and pleasurable?

I often look to my Celtic lineage as a way of relearning how to be at home in my body. I remember a feeling of profound delight when I happened upon the idea of *Cynefin*. *Cynefin* is Welsh and refers to a place where you feel you belong and where the nature around you feels right and welcoming. *Cynefin* (pronounced ki-NEH-vin) cannot be directly translated into English, but it is commonly translated as 'habitat' and means a place of multiple belongings. *Cynefin* encompasses the reality that every person is rooted in multiple pasts that we bring to bear in the now. This kind of belonging allows us to fully sensitize to the world around us and inhabit space as our whole selves.

As a creative and artist, I aim to always cultivate a sense of *Cynefin* in my work, in my studio, in my body, and in my space-holding. For me, *Cynefin* means "true home" or to be truly seen or witnessed in a physical setting. It invokes a kind of deep self-permission. This is the kind of belonging I want to explore as we tap into our senses and step into Beltane season.

## INCUBATION

Any embodiment practice begins with breath. It is connected to every organ in our body. Our ability to control our breath or release control of our breath is often an indicator of what the body is experiencing at any moment. The breath is a bellwether for the body. It is also a primary point of focus as we begin to understand how our bodies perceive and receive information.

I want you to think back to your child self. Barring a medical respiratory challenge, no one had to teach you how to breathe. It was autonomic. When you nursed or drank from a bottle, you quickly mastered the art of taking turns between breath and gulp. When you ran, your body took in as much air as it needed. When you shouted or sang, you didn't have to consciously manage your airflow. The sound simply came rushing out of you, clear and inexhaustible. I want us to renew our relationship with that uncultivated wild breath and the undomesticated nature of our original lung capacity.

In her book *Gardening at the Dragon's Gate,* master gardener and Zen practitioner Wendy Johnson writes that "there is very little true wilderness remaining in the modern world. And yet wildness persists. It endures underneath the paved-over pathways of our cities as well as on the fringe of urban farmland. It persists in patches, sumps, and wallows, in weedy tangles everywhere on Earth."

The ideas that Wendy shares here about the botanical world could also be said of the human heart. Each one of us has undergone a kind of domestication process that began in earnest upon our birth. This process also served to edit and hem in our voice (breath). Tapping into the power of the uncultivated world is key to unlearning some of our domestication. Here are some questions to consider as you write in your journal or draw in your sketchbook this season:

What does the "uncultivated world" feel, smell, and sound like to you?

What permissions do you find there?

And how are you staying in relationship to the uncultivated world as you inhabit domesticated land?

Where, in spite of society's efforts to domesticate you, do you find wildness in yourself? In your body? In your heart? In your voice?

ACTION

When we tend to the altar of our bodies, when we begin to unhook from centuries of domestication, when we begin to breathe the free air of self-expression, our authentic selves start to bloom and show up with more frequency. One of the ways you might experience this authentic unfolding is through a heightened sense of connection to the sights, smells, and sounds around you. I like to engage this newfound perceptive power by taking a sensory tour of my home or garden. It's a way to reintroduce myself to my surroundings. I call it "creative puttering."

Creative puttering is one of my favorite and joy-inducing embodiment practices. I consider it both a form of authentic discovery and mental rest. The byproduct is often an increase in creative flow. Most people categorize puttering as time spent in aimless activity or in less approving circles, looking busy while not doing much. But creative puttering is an absolute pleasure. There is no goal or aim in mind and it requires you to stop concentrating.

The magic of puttering happens when your mind is at ease and free to float from one pleasant thought to the next. At the same time, puttering involves mild physical activity. It keeps you physically moving at an unhurried pace while you're busy with small tasks.

In this way, puttering does not mimic traditional meditation. We generally sit still to meditate. Instead, puttering requires that you maintain a level of activity, using your body to perform little tasks that require minimal physical and mental exertion. Creative puttering is my way of practicing patience while waiting for my senses to sharpen. It's all about letting go of deadlines, expectations for results, and yearnings for achievement. Sounds pretty good, right?

If you're someone who learns better when they're moving and physically interacting with whatever they're focused on, then you'll love creative puttering. You might even already do this naturally, but I like to set aside time in my calendar for this practice. This is a way to re-tune my perceptions and allow my surroundings to communicate with me.

Here's how I do it: At the beginning of each week I take a look at my schedule and identify an open hour, preferably after I've completed my important "have-to" tasks for the day. This usually occurs for me sometime between my last appointment and making dinner. Other times, this happens on a weekend morning when I don't have a busy day ahead of me. Once I've identified a good time, I block it out and write in "creative puttering".

Then, when the time comes, I make something lovely to drink and pick out some music to suit my mood. (Joni Mitchel and Lauren Hill are my go-to artists for creative puttering.) Music playing and yummy libation at the ready, I walk around my house, garden, or studio noticing what's out, what's dirty, what's unfinished, what's growing, and what needs tending. I'm not engaging yet. I just notice.

After I've made the rounds, something will call to me. An unread newspaper clipping, a stack of books that need to be shelved, a sad looking plant that needs hydration, or an out of place chair that longs to be placed in another part of the house. It begins as a loose form of tidying up without judgment, as if I'm making space for something else. But the 'something else' has yet to show itself.

Soon the clutter-clearing shifts and I can feel an urge for something more focused, as if my mind is an iris that is closing in around the pupil. The shift occurs when my body settles and my mind has released its hold on creating an "outcome." This moment of embodied shift takes practice. You may not feel it the first or second time you try creative puttering. But eventually, your inner hum will become detectable. You'll sense it.

Flow state is sacred. And creative puttering is just one of many ways that I invite flow state into my life. Once this transition has occurred, I ask myself what am I craving? What needs to be nourished or tended to? Then I follow that voice.

My creative puttering can turn towards a variety of cravings. It might look like letter writing, or collecting pine cones, or creating a collage, or weeding, or reading through an old box of Christmas cards, or photographing sunlight as it plays on my windowsill. But sometimes it transforms into big creative and emotional breakthroughs. Either way, this practice of puttering without a goal is deeply nourishing to my soul. It is a simple practice that invites me into a deeper relationship with my perceptive powers and authentic yearnings. And even if all I do is tidy up my desk, it produces a sense of space and joy.

## INTEGRATION

The spell we are casting this season is one in service of the senses. The ancient Celts were rooted in the conviction that each soul possesses within it a wisdom that comes directly from our inter-relatedness to the Earth and that this is a sacred relationship based on embodied listening. Right now, we humans seem to be suffering from a kind of soul-forgetfulness. May our creative work be a song for collective remembering, a seed planted in the soil of our authentic selves.

All thriving – physical, spiritual, and creative – begins with a seed. The miraculous nature of a seed is that it contains the entirety of both its past and future. It transmits potent information about time, place, memory, and possibility. But the seed, for all its potential, must receive certain stimuli if it is to fulfill its mission: warmth, light, water, nutrients, and healthy soil. Your creative work needs these things too. Here are some questions for your journal:

**How are you tending your creative garden at this time? What practices do you have or would you like to have in place to ensure growth and thriving?**

**What seeds are you planting? Which ideas have you set in motion and how are you empowering them to take root?**

**What nutrients are you turning into the soil of your life / garden / creativity?**

As we expand on the seed and garden metaphor for our creative work, let's consider how we might deepen our embodiment practice as a form of deep noticing and remembering. If the seed can transmit information about its past, present, and future, then perhaps its root, flower and fruit can share the secrets of its longevity, lineage, and love. We can strengthen our creative connection to ancestral knowledge by seeking mentorship and apprenticeship from plants. Are there plants in your garden or elsewhere that you would like to intentionally court and apprentice yourself? Let's consider how you might go about this apprenticeship.

**Which seeds and plants can be found in your part of the world? Do you know their names? Which seeds and plants did your near and distant ancestors live in relationship with? What traditional foods were harvested from their gardens and cooked in their kitchens? Do you have a relationship with those original plant and food allies? Do some research about the food traditions from your lineage. This can be both tied to your chosen family or by DNA. What do they have to teach you? And in what ways are you listening?**

**Pick one plant or herb in your area or one that was tended by your ancestors, and learn everything you can about it. Would it be possible to grow it yourself? How might you include it in your diet or daily rituals?**

The Arrowleaf Balsamroot is always the first flower to appear on the heels of the Eastern Oregon snow melt. It's wildly abundant during Beltane season and its presence announces the pending arrival of a host of other native plants. Its sage-colored leaves have a fuzzy texture and the bloom is a bright yellow-orange with a dark center. Nearly all parts of this plant were used as food by various indigenous tribes: the roots, stems, leaves, flowers, and seeds all have nutritional and medicinal qualities. This is notable since it's the first flower to appear on the scene after the deep winter freeze.

Let's imagine ourselves as medicinal plants. We have roots that connect us to our purpose and lineage. We have stems that hold us up when the winds begin to blow. Our leaves are wide and open to receive the gifts of sunlight, capable of alchemy and transformation. And our creative expression is a kind of flower that blooms and unfolds when the conditions are right.

**When your roots are harvested and consumed, how do they heal the body?**

**What alchemizes in the system when your stems are steeped in a nourishing broth?**

**When your leaves are crushed into a poultice and applied to the skin, what relief does it offer?**

**When your petals are dried for tea and imbibed, what magical properties are released?**

**What unique medicine do you offer the world?**

**Pull out your sketchbook, and use the line-drawing techniques from the previous chapter to make a botanical study of yourself as a medicinal plant. You can even label all of the parts of your plant-self.**

### ONE-WORD PROMPTS FOR BELTANE

Pollinate • Pleasure • Bloom • Body • Sensitize
Marriage • Efflorescence • Generate • Domesticate • Wild
Kiss • Belong • Echo • Petal • Limit
Flourish • Intimate • Heart • Apprentice • Fertile
Lilac • Midwife • Moss • Paradise • Imbibe
Song • Earth • Uncultivated • Radiant • Mother

### THE NEXT SIX WEEKS

The painter Agnes Martin said, "The development of sensibility is the most important thing for children and adults alike, but is much more possible for children.... Adults are very busy, taught to run all the time. You cannot run and be very aware of your inspirations." This season, slow down. Stop running. Use the prompts in this chapter to awaken your senses, coax your authentic self out into the open and become more aware of your inspirations.

The time between Beltane and the summer solstice is a little over 6 weeks. This is the season for radical self-love and creative pollination. Get low and listen for the crackling sound of leaves unfurling and petals popping free of their buds. Connect with the plants around you, carve out time for creative puttering, and carry your journal and sketchbook wherever you go. Then when you see or hear or feel something stir, you can catch it and scribble it down. Let's search for mushrooms, lollygag in the garden, and luxuriate in the lap of mama Earth. Inspiration is everywhere. (And when you have a moment, look up the original meaning of the word lollygag. Sexy season just got a whole lot sexier.)

### CROSS THE THRESHOLD

Before we transition through the gates of Beltane into the activism and energy of the summer solstice, I want to address an obstacle that may prevent us from a nourishing and effective embodiment practice: comparison. When it comes to my body, Sonya Renee Taylor is one of my greatest teachers. I once heard her speak about her book *The Body Is Not An Apology*, and she said, "If I am comparing myself to others, I am accepting a framework of hierarchy — a hierarchy that says some bodies are better than others." If I am comparing myself to others, I am taking my place as a rung on the ladder of hierarchy. My participation in this hierarchy, no matter where on the ladder I exist, requires some people to be below me. This self-selecting process is a textbook tool for oppressors.

When I wish myself different, compare myself to others, or allow domestication, colonization, and negative messages to influence my sense of self-love, I am not embodying my true self. Nor am I in alignment with my work as a creator. But when I step outside the machine and refuse to take my place on the ladder of hierarchy, I disrupt the system that says some bodies are better than others. I disrupt ableism, fat-phobia, racism, sexism, homophobia and transphobia. Pow! Thank you, Sonya Renee Taylor.

Radical self-love, which requires a rejection of comparison, is a key part of dismantling interlocking oppressive structures that keep us all separate, desperate, and strangers to our natural state of belonging. Separate from our natural state of *Cynefin*: true home.

Belonging is at the core of our work within *The Creative Alchemy Cycle*. My mission as an artist and storyteller is to draw us closer into right-relationship. And that can only happen when we radically, shamelessly love ourselves. It happens when we treat the body as altar and pay obeisance to what we really feel, see, hear, and think. We can step off the ladder. We can create a new world. We can be whole.

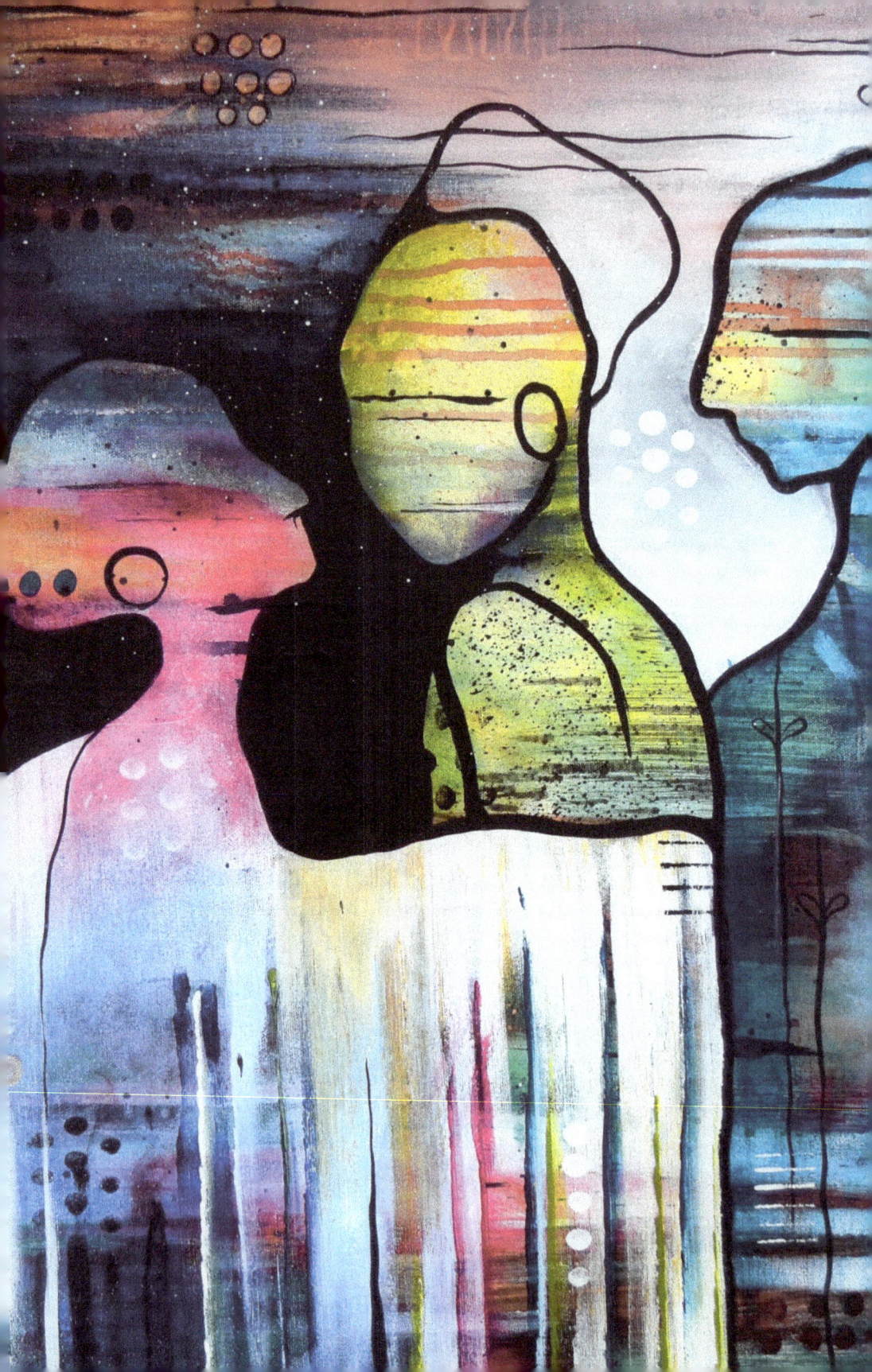

# 5

# WE ARE FIRE: LITHA

## ACTIVIST PRACTICE

**The Call:** Our liberation is bound together.

**The Question:** How do I use my innate creative gifts to take action?

**The Time:** June 19th - 22nd

**The Origin:** Litha (pronounced LI-tha), also known as the summer solstice, marks the longest day of the year. The Druids called midsummer *Alban Hefin*, which translates to "light of the summer." Litha, which also means light, is a festival dedicated to the life-giving, regenerative powers of the sun.

**The Imagery:** Fire, Sun, Chrysalis

**The Themes:** Creative Risk, Focus, Discernment, and Activism

SUN-WORSHIPPERS, THIS IS YOUR MOMENT. SUMMER SOLSTICE, CALLED Litha on the Celtic calendar, marks the longest day of the year. In the northern hemisphere, Litha falls between June 19th and 22nd. Since it is the peak of the solar year, with the sun at the height of its life-giving power, the *Creative Alchemy Cycle* asks that we consider our own power. Let's explore the places where our creative practice moves into activism. And for our purposes, an activist is someone who uses their unique gifts or talents to work in service of political or social change.

Prentis Hemphill, a somatic therapist and activist who came to prominence during the Black Lives Matter movement, refers to something they call "touching the dream," which is the idea that we are practicing in real time the future we wish to bring into existence. It's those moments when we feel, in our bodies, the reality of our dreams being made manifest. That is "touching the dream." And most times, it only happens in small doses: a second, a moment.

The stories, thoughts, and prompts I offer in this chapter are not prescriptive. We all have our own way into this work. I am a student and practitioner, not a source of theory, history, or leadership. Leadership comes from those on the front lines of their movements. Those of us who stand with them are here to center their words and work, with the understanding that with deep listening, it might inform our own analysis and activism. My hope is that this chapter invites you into a deeper relationship with your own values and serves as permission to use your creative process as a catalyst for justice. Let's practice touching the dream together.

CALLING YOU HOME – A SEASONAL HOMILY FOR LITHA

"But how will I make money?" Earning potential was the first and sometimes only concern people would share with me and Jack, my former partner of 20 years, about our decision to move from Dallas, Texas to rural Eastern Oregon. And I suppose it's a fair question, since we've been trained from an early age to center income as the chief identifier of a "good decision."

Jack was climbing the ladder as a tenured professor in corporate academia and I was working as many jobs as possible to fill in our financial gaps. We were right where America wanted us: working long hours, begging the state for health care for our medically fragile child, chasing down paper-work, slowly drowning under an expanding mortgage we couldn't really afford, dependent on the big box stores for our daily needs, isolated from our community based on class and access, and watching the city's wealth gap get larger and larger as we stretched ourselves thinner and thinner.

Our decision to move seemed romantic to some and downright reckless to others. One of my partner's colleagues referred to our move as "escaping the velvet cage". Her comment was apt and illuminated a startling truth: we were trapped, all of us, in an extractive system that used up all our gifts and talents in exchange for a certain level of perceived comfort. But once we woke up to this reality, we knew we had to disengage. The health and mental well-being of our entire family was in jeopardy. And we knew there had to be a better way.

Pine Valley is situated at the base of the Wallowa Whitman mountain range, the largest expanse of unincorporated wilderness in the lower 48 states. It is rural with a capital 'R'. We knew this move would require that we sell off many of our belongings and lighten our load. But it also required that we take a long hard look at how we thought of ourselves. Who were we without our jobs and connections? Would we be able to shed outdated identities that were tied to our status, our work-life, and our little slice of perceived social capital?

My first few months in our new home turned out to be a roller-coaster of big feelings. And the question that greeted me every morning was "Who am I now?" I was still trying to be all the things that I was before the move. I was still checking my phone 47 times a day. I was still hooked up to a culture that said if I wasn't hustling 24/7, then I was lazy, behind, uninformed, a liability.

My new environment was a paradise. It was quiet. Creeks flowed freely. I could hear coyotes at night. Main street closed at 6pm. Rushing a conversation was seen by locals as rude. And a million stars burned silently overhead, unencumbered by light-bleed. Why couldn't I unhook and release? I know now that I was feeling the residual trauma of grind culture. It's a powerful capitalistic tool used for a trifecta of purposes: to maximize labor, oppress marginalized communities, and all while making the hustle and grind a social signifier of importance. As my new natural surroundings began to work its slow magic, I began to awaken from the spell. And when you begin to wake up, you can finally see clearly that the entire apparatus is a supremacy system. And I was a part of it.

We had been living in our new home for five months when I was offered some summer work on a thinning and harvest crew at Eagle Creek Orchard. The summer solstice was only a few weeks away and all of the local fruit trees were leafing out with a sense of urgency. For all of Earth's plants and creatures, nothing is so fundamental as the length of the day. All rhythms, all growth, all living and dying, rests upon its axis and strength. The orchard was no different. I had never done this kind of work before but I was excited to connect with area farmers and participate in the stewardship and care of our most local food source. Plus I really like peaches.

Robert Cordtz, the orchardist and owner, was a gracious and willing teacher. On my first day he handed me a pair of Japanese thinning shears. The rubbery red handles felt solid in my hand. Robert drew my attention to the razor sharp steel blades. "Careful with these," he said. "They'll bite cha."

We started in the Asian Pear block with a variety called Shinseiki. Robert explained that my job was to use the shears to snip off most of the fruit. This seemed like a murderous instruction. Robert found a tightly bound group of baby fruit. "Look", he said. "There are eight pears all fruiting together in the same place. Find the one that looks the healthiest, usually the king blossom right in the middle, and cut away everything around it."

"Everything?" I asked?

Rob smiled. "Everything. It needs space, air, and the support of the branch. If we keep all of the fruit, the branch will break under the weight."

The morning was clear and cold. I could hear calves in the neighboring field calling for their first meal of the day. I unhooked the rubber band that secured the shears in a closed position and approached the tree. I gazed at the nearest branch and saw that it overwhlemed with fruit. Every spring blossom had been pollinated. I started at the end and worked my way towards the trunk. By the time I reached the middle of the tree, I had dropped 90 percent of the fruit on the orchard floor. I could feel the hard balls of potential food under my boots like marbles. My shoulders dropped. I began to breathe with the tree. And I know this sounds crazy, but I felt the tree relax. She had been sending all of her love and sugar stores to every single piece of fruit, a mad frenzy of spring-time life-energy. And when I cut away the burden of overproduction, the tree straightened up and let out a sigh of gratitude.

Robert and I made our way around the tree until her trim was complete. I gestured to the ground and asked about the fruit heaped around the roots. "I guess we've made quite a mess. Should I rake it up?" I asked.

"No way!" said Robert. "It has a new job to do."

"What's that?"

"Feed the soil," he replied.

I had spent my entire life thinking that it was my job to do it all: make the plan, create the art, lead the way, save the world. But no one does this work alone. And no one gets a prize for pretending that they can. When we're under the societal spell that says we have to constantly produce, we become complicit in the very harm from which we suffer.

Mercy came to us both that day, me and the pear tree. When we have the courage to cut away our need to know it all and do it all, what we release might become fuel for something else – something generative. What a gift. What a chance.

Lighten the load.
Toss the excess.
Disentangle.
Strip down.
Use the shears.
Rest your limbs.
And above all,
wake up.

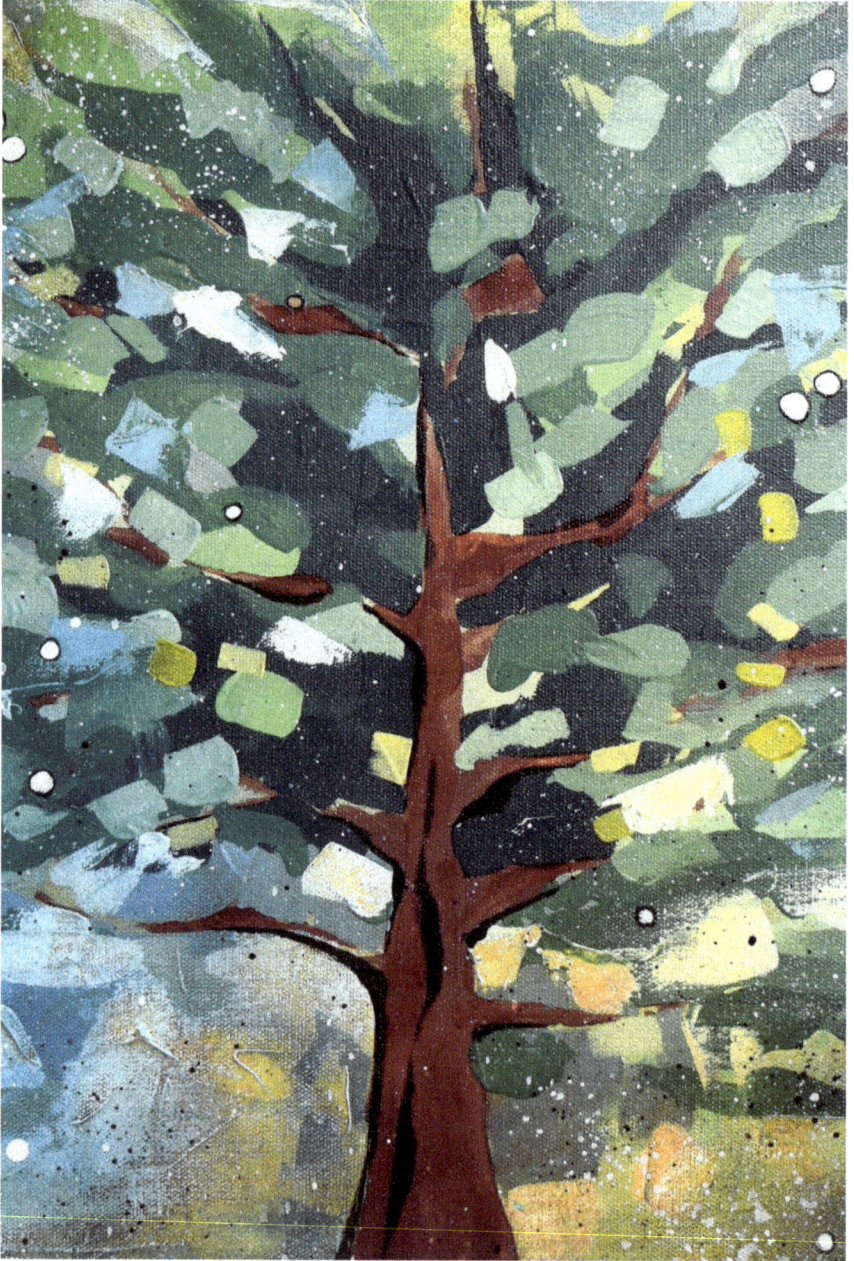

## Tend the Altar

Hells Canyon lies about fifteen minutes to the east of my home in Pine Valley. This is the time of year when mother nature turns up the heat and Hells Canyon really earns its name. It was a bright day in late June. A Canyon Wren lighted, weightless on the limb of the Elm tree near my front door. I heard his whistle first, a descending melody with tumbling notes that sound like an echo. Then I saw him, rusty red-brown and handsome with a gleaming cream-colored throat that bounced as he sang. A bird watcher friend tells me that these wrens are native to Hells Canyon and they nest in tiny holes along the steep, rocky cliff walls of the Snake River. The bird sang again, hopped along the Elm branch, dismounted and landed on my neighbor's fence. He listened. *Piu, piu, piu, piu,* he called again. And then I heard it. Another bird joined his song. Then another. And then other birds joined in. I heard the Robin and the Chickadee and a Warbler and somewhere a Magpie squawked. It was quite a cacophony. The wren seemed pleased.

The Canyon Wren is a fairly common bird, but I don't usually see them. They're pretty elusive in town and prefer to spend their time at home among the cliffs. There are also environmental factors. A decade of spring heat waves have killed their offspring while still in the nests. But here he was, this beautiful brown bird, out shouting in the streets. Tiny bird. Big voice.

## Altar Practice

This season, let's invite some other voices into the altar process and make it a community affair. It's easy to ignore the tune of the Canyon Wren when he sings alone. It's much harder when he's joined by a chorus. Since your altar is a place of concentrated energy and intention, opening your altar to the larger community is a way to practice shared power. There is a vital resonance between our private altars and our public offers.

The easiest and most immediate way to open up your altar is to include images and words of those you seek to learn from. This year, I created an altar devoted to disability justice in preparation for my work as a facilitator with the board of a medical health foundation. My altar included a favorite quote from activist Mia Mingus, a copy of *Care Work* by Leah Lakshmi Piepzna-Samarasinha, and a photo of my son Charlie who experiences Cerebral Palsy and Epilepsy. In this way, I invoked the words of disability justice warriors, energetically centered the stories of those on the front lines, and made it personal with my own connections.

Sometimes communal altar opportunities will happen spontaneously. For instance, a few years ago, I helped establish a learning garden at a very diverse public school in an under-resourced community in Dallas, Texas. Many of the students were also children of undocumented laborers and refugees. Twelve different languages were spoken on campus. The garden served as a source of plant education, food sovereignty, and land stewardship, but it also provided a neutral gathering place outside the classroom. Nature, like music, was a language that everyone understood. The teachers and students chose an elevated flat rock in a central location to share exciting found objects from the garden: leaves, rocks, seed pods, insect husks, etc. Soon it took on a life of its own and children began to bring things from home to place on the altar – a family trinket, a trading card from their home country, a small toy. It was clear that this was a powerful way to share a piece of themselves with the larger community. Every day, children would gather around the rock to share stories about the objects they'd contributed to the impromptu altar, and in doing so, bridged cultural gaps and strengthened their personal bonds.

The garden altar was spontaneous, but we can also be more intentional. Potlucks are a beautiful way to share responsibility for a communal meal. But we can up the ante and ask everyone to bring an object of importance and reverence. Invite guests to arrange their objects in the middle of the dinner table. Light a candle. Then, as a kind of collective prayer, take a few moments for each guest to share a brief story of their chosen object. In this way, all voices are heard and each person offers a bit of their own story. Breaking bread together in this way can also be a source of healing and communicating across difference.

One of my favorite communal altars was built by strangers in a boardroom during a social justice conference. Our facilitator was theater artist and activist Daniel Banks. Al Green was playing on the speakers as each participant entered the room. Daniel greeted us, invited us to choose a dry erase marker of any color, and asked us to write our answer to the question, "What is an ally?" We danced our way to the whiteboard (it's impossible *not* to dance to Al Green) and shared our thoughts in all of the colors of the rainbow. The workshop commenced against the backdrop of our words – "co-conspirator, risk-taker, advocate, accomplice, catalyst" –  and like a stained glass window in a sanctuary, it took on a special kind of glow. At the end of our time together, we formed a semicircle around the whiteboard and sang the hymn "Guide My Feet."

Intention can transform anything into an altar. And an altar is a place to practice power. Making it communal is a potent way to build community, uplift each voice in the room, and center the lived-experiences of those for and with whom you are advocating.

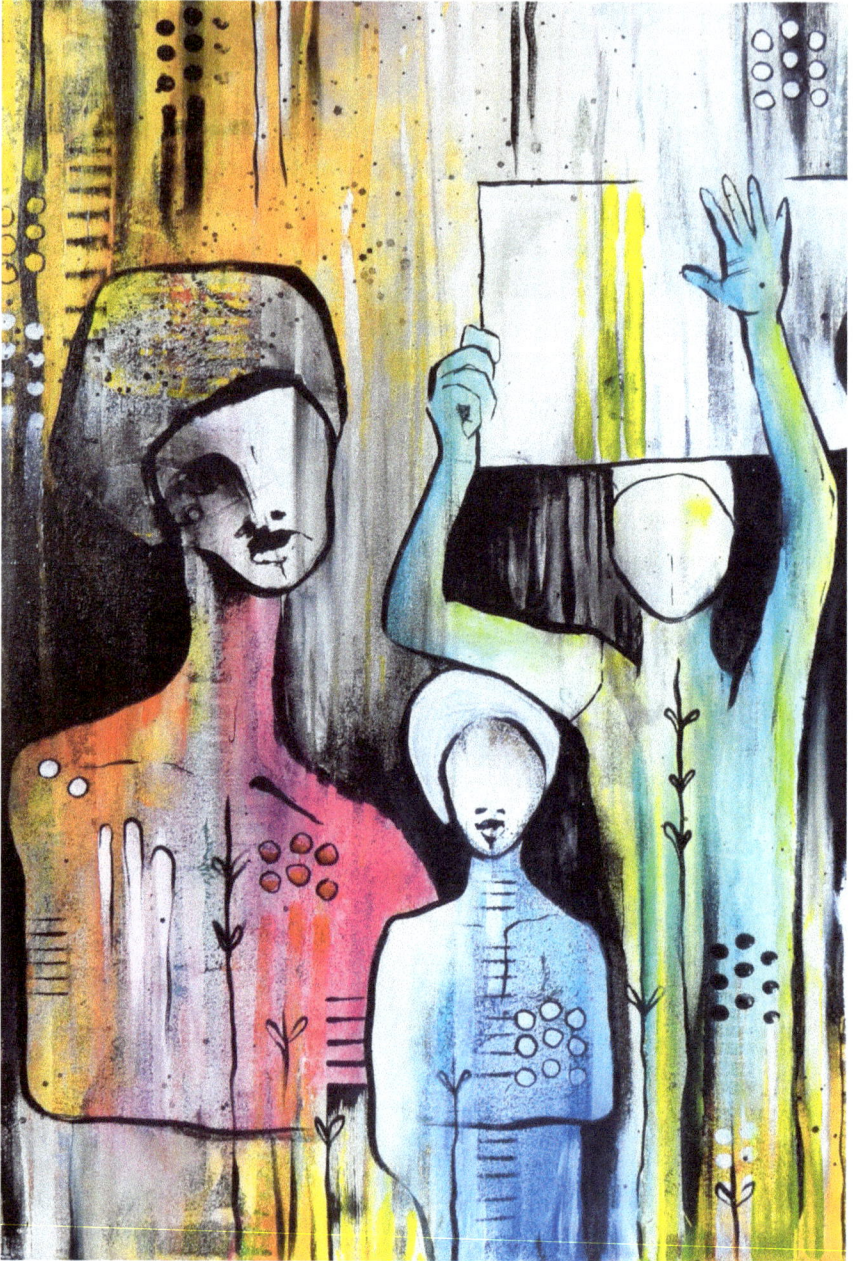

ACTIVIST PRACTICE

In college I studied creative writing, gender studies, and theater. I took all sorts of mind-opening classes about Theatre of the Oppressed and the Harlem Renaissance and intersectional feminism and the Black Arts Movement. It was during this time that I was also introduced to community organizing and social justice work. I owe my life and work to the many queer Black femmes at Mills College who called me in, lovingly handed my ass to me in our gender studies class, and baptized me with the writings of bell hooks, Audre Lorde, Cherríe Moraga, and June Jordan. They opened my eyes to the divine nature of right-relationship, asked potent questions, and transformed the trajectory of my life as an artist, change-maker, and activist. It was the beginning of an awakening that continues to this day.

Author and activist Gloria Anzaldúa tells us to "Write with your eyes like painters, with your ears like musicians, with your feet like dancers. You are the truthsayer with quill and torch. Write with your tongues on fire... put your shit on the paper." Or rather, since we're also talking about activism, "Put your shit on the line." Let's take some risks.

This also brings to mind Joy Harjo's words: "I am the throat of the mountains, a night wind who burns with every breath she takes." As the solstice sun turns up the dial and draws us out into the streets to sing our songs, I am holding Anzaldúa's and Harjo's words close and meditating on what it means to have a "tongue on fire" – to be the "throat of the mountains." I live along the edge of the Pacific Rim, which is dotted with inactive volcanoes to the west and Hells Canyon, our country's deepest gorge, to the east. At their core, these geological wonders are a pathway to Earth's surface for molten rock. They breathe fire. This is the image I am invoking for our work this season.

Speak truth. Be a conduit for stories that scald and art that scorches. Sing like the Canyon Wren so that your tune tumbles into the air and ignites the songs of others. Burn with every breath. Let's do as Rumi recommends and set our lives on fire. Who are we saving it for? Let our work in the world be combustible, fuel for our next bold move.

## Incubation

Chrysalis and butterfly imagery permeates my art. I love their beauty, the miraculous nature of their existence, and the expressive emergence they represent. While the butterfly exudes the triumphant, visible, outer transformation, the cocoon encapsulates the private internal process. And for the chrysalis, there is also a darker, deeper message: that for life to change, we must also change ourselves. Social justice work is all about transformation. And transformation requires that we surrender.

The work of waking up to the world around us and answering the call of our particular time is chrysalis work. It requires that we trust the wisdom of our bodies as we deconstruct ourselves, liquify our former structure, and build back better. As we prepare our creative altar and light the fires of our purpose-driven work, remember that your voice matters. What you see, how you see it, and the sense-making you craft out of that seeing is the gift you have to give.

You are being called to step into the center of your power right now. And while you may be hesitant, you know more than you think you know. While your readiness may not feel like confidence, this is the moment to pump up the balloon of your belief, hang on with conviction, and allow your feet to leave the ground.

Remember that you don't have to *be* confident to *practice* confidence. Practice definitely comes first. So try it on and see how it feels.

Chest open.
Arms wide.
Chin up.
Lift off.

∼

On April 29, 1992, I watched as Los Angeles news outlets broadcast videos of violence erupting in South Los Angeles on the heels of the Rodney King verdict. Like so many others, I followed the case closely and saw the footage of police officers beating the breath out of King.

Mayor Tom Bradley denounced the ruling and said "The jury's verdict will never blind the world to what we saw on the videotape."

I was fourteen years old at the time and didn't know what to do with my rage. The jury acquitted all four officers of any wrong-doing. Like most white children, I had been kept ignorant of the realities facing my Black peers. My shock was real, but it was also evidence of my privilege. I didn't have the language for any of this at the time. My English teacher suggested that I take my feelings to the page and write something. While I had been journaling since the age of twelve, this was the first time I remember intentionally using art to transform my confusion and anger into something generative.

The act of taking our sorrow, pain, or rage to the page is not in and of itself a form of activism. Rather it is a tool for self-awareness, a way to sharpen our analysis of what we see and experience. It is an incubatory process and a great place to begin. Here are some questions to take to your journal:

**When was the first time you employed art as a tool to manage big feelings? You may have been very young or it may have been last month.**

**How did your creative engagement manifest? Perhaps you wrote a poem or a song. Perhaps you went for a walk and collected stones along your path. Perhaps you made a collage or a nourishing meal.**

**How did you feel afterwards?**

~

Creativity reveals itself in many ways. Of course you can make a painting, write a poem, or take to the stage. But the creative impulse also arrives when we arrange a vase of flowers, write a letter, love well, plant bulbs in the fall for our spring garden, or collect fallen leaves for an impromptu mandala along the sidewalk.

**When was the very first time you realized that you were a creative**

**force, capable of bringing forth your own vision? This may be a moment you now realize looking back. You may have been very young, or it may have been much later in life. How did this newfound creative power make you feel and how did it change the way you moved through the world?**

## ACTION

Here's what I know for sure: our liberation is bound together. It is interconnected, interdependent, and collective. There are no saviors here, only accomplices. The poet Audre Lorde reminds us that, "I am not free while any woman is unfree, even when her shackles are very different from my own." Every successful historical movement for social change was buoyed by networks of intentional, interwoven collective action. This doesn't mean you have to be in the thick of the protest or fighting it out in the eye of the storm. But it does mean you have to be responsive to the needs of the community, prepared to take informed action within your chosen sphere. It means that you understand that your own ability to be free is connected to the freedom of others. Your freedom is my freedom.

One of the most potent things we can do for our advocacy and activism is to identify our role(s) as change-makers and justice-minded creatives. As a creative who weaves together art and activism, I am called to look my time squarely in the eye and ask 'What is mine to do?' We all have a role to play. And we all have tools at our disposal to disrupt the status quo and co-envision a new way forward. But sometimes we don't realize that we have access to these tools, or that they're even ours to use. The singer and activist Nina Simone once said, "I have to constantly re-identify myself to myself, reactivate my own standards, my own convictions about what I'm doing and why." This kind of inquiry was core to Nina's music and mission. And it is also part of my process.

What is uniquely yours to do? For some of us, this can be a difficult question to answer. And that's okay. Part of the work of the *Creative Alchemy Cycle* is allowing your purpose-driven work to surface. This takes time and introspection.

My own activism manifests in a variety of ways, and changes depending on who I'm with and what's needed. I'm a white, queer, low-income mother of a child experiencing disability, living in one of the most rural parts of the United States. I can't really take to the streets. And I don't have a large sweeping audience to mobilize through social media. So, I must get creative and weave my activism into my offerings, my writing, my parenting, my partnerships, my rural community organizing, my one-on-one interactions, and into the very fabric of how I manage my business as a solo artist. These are the places where I have influence.

Where do you have influence? What are your particular talents, competencies, and resources? Activist and social strategist Deepa Iyer writes, "In our lives and as part of movements and organizations, many of us play different roles in pursuit of equity, shared liberation, inclusion, and justice. And yet, we often get lost and confused, or we are newcomers to ongoing social change efforts and don't know where to start, or we are catalyzed into action in the midst of a crisis in our community." I want us to think about ways in which we can contribute to the success of social change in a way that is aligned with who we are as individuals and creators. Please know that we can inhabit many roles and that our roles can change depending on the needs of our community, who we're working with, and our capacity for engagement.

Perhaps you're a bard or storyteller, re-shaping histories and sharing community stories in a way that shifts the dominant cultural narrative. Or maybe your gifts lie in mutual care models, where you can nourish, feed, and tend to the wellbeing of the community. Or perhaps you are a detail-oriented person who delights in organizing resources and shaping the message. And for those of us who don't know where to begin, do as Mr. Rogers says and look for the helpers. Seek out the people who are already working in the spheres you feel called to and use your creative gifts to uplift and amplify their great work.

Here are some questions to consider and journal about:

Have you ever considered your creative gifts as integral to movements for social change?

As you think about your talents, gifts, and resources, are there any that immediately feel transferable?

How might your values and gifts come together in service of the things you most care about?

Expand your idea of community beyond humans to the more-than-human world. How can you leverage your creative gifts in service to plants, animals, water, land?

Where do you have access where others may not? And how might you redistribute excess resources?

How can you weave together your access and your creative gifts as a tool for social change?

*For more information about identifying your role(s) in social justice movements check out Deepa Iyer's Social Change Ecosystem Map or Joanna Macy's "roles and responsibilities" for The Work That Reconnects. You'll find their work and more in the index.*

## A Manifesto

Every good revolutionist has a manifesto. Declarative statements are good for the soul, especially when they are an outer reflection of your inner values. Are there causes you believe in? Are there people you'd walk into fire for? Are there things for which you'd put your body on the line? There comes a time when you need to tap your internal moral compass and express it outwardly. Showing up for others in a space of authentic allyship is an important part of building beloved community. And this kind of action always involves risk. Welcome it. Tell people you love them. Show up when they need you most. Get on the phone and call your representative. Speak up at that

PTA meeting. Or, if you are called forth by your community, lead the charge. Whatever you do - do it out loud.

As a tangible way to express core values and practices, my friend and mentor Anya Hankin asks all of her clients to create what she calls a "Leadership Humxnifesto." It was under her guidance that I created mine. My leadership manifesto has been a vital way to continue to show up in my wholeness with my core values at top of mind. In fact, I re-read it every time I'm about to step into a room as a facilitator or guide.

This is my Leadership Humxnifesto:

* * * My leadership trusts the collective wisdom of the community and delights in its unfolding.

* * * My leadership is informed by movements for racial justice and is rooted in storytelling traditions from my Celtic lineage.

* * * My leadership is in symbiotic relationship with Earth's natural cycles and is expressed as eco-spiritualism.

* * * My leadership challenges white supremacy by rejecting perfectionism, centering BIPOC voices, and practicing robust accountability and reparations.

* * * My leadership contributes to a legacy of matriarchal wisdom and uplifts creativity as a primary tool for healing ourselves and our planet.

* * * My leadership lays paving stones on the path to collective liberation.

* * * My leadership feels like home, love, permission.

**Let's write our manifesto! (Or maybe yours will be a femifesto, or an ecofesto, or a humanifesto.) Choose a focus for your activism. My**

**example above centered leadership. What will yours be? Yours could be a Healing Manifesto, a Creative Manifesto, a Care Manifesto, a Solidarity Manifesto, a Love Manifesto. (You get the idea.) What will be the focus of your manifesto?**

Now that you've chosen a focus, think about how you want to get it down on paper. You can create bullet points as I did above or you can write in long-form paragraphs. You can make a cluster map in your sketchbook with your focus at the center and each facet as a spoke of a wheel. You can write an entire book! Make it work for you. Here are some prompts to get you started:

**What does your leadership, healing, care, creativity, etc. do? What does it create, contribute, build, acknowledge, uplift, liberate, amplify, know, catalyze, facilitate, trust, tend, inspire, or challenge? Where does it come from? What is its lineage? What is it informed by? And what does it feel like?**

Your manifesto is a wonderful tool for grounding into a sense of purpose. It's also a way to check back in with yourself and ask, "How am I using my innate gifts to take action in alignment with my values?" Your manifestos will change as you do. This is a lovely exercise to come back to year after year. And you can make more than one! I have one for my business, one for my family, and one for my leadership.

∼

Sometimes activism is not an act of *doing*, but an act of *not* doing. When my partner and I left our jobs in the city and moved to rural Oregon we were, in essence, saying no. No to extractive work. No to transactional relationships. No to capital earned through oppressive structures. No to false comfort. And no to our complicity and participation in systems that oppressed ourselves and others. This was especially important to us as a white family.

If we are to successfully dismantle supremacy systems we must divest from the benefits they afford us. If we are consciously or unconsciously leveraging white-body privilege (or trading on our thinness, or banking on our physical ability or placing our inherent worth in our neuro-typicalness) then we are perpetuating harm. We must betray the privilege of our unearned advantages, whatever they may be, and interrupt supremacy systems by refusing to be their beneficiary.

We also have to get clear about what we want to create. One of my stated goals as an artist and activist (as you read in my manifesto) is to lay paving stones on our path to collective liberation. I'm also committed to right-relationship, which compels me to disrupt supremacy systems. I want to contribute to a culture where everyone is able to claim belonging for themselves and be the agent of their own freedom and growth. I am only one person and I am also an imperfect vessel for this work, but my hope is that if white folks like me speak openly about race and the nightmare of white dominance with other white folks, we can practice our work for right-relationship in real time. This is intricately connected to my creative work and I believe it is a viable pathway for healing the wounds of our disconnection.

Divestment and disruption can come in many forms. And we can use our creative tools to interrogate our privilege and interrupt harm. This kind of activist practice might manifest in the following ways:

Stop talking and listen with the intent to learn and change your behavior.

Elevate the practice of accountability as a holy artform, rather than something to be avoided. Parents, we can practice this in real time in our homes as a way of normalizing accountability and repair work for our children. As we become practiced in small ways, we can develop a culture of accountability in our communities as well. (More about this in the next chapter.)

Show up in solidarity with the people leading justice movements in your area. Work alongside them. You are not a hero. There is not a group of people out there awaiting rescue. That is saviorism and counterproductive for liberation movements. And again, stop talking and listen with the intent to learn.

Break cycles of socialization that pass white supremacy or any supremacy system down generationally. This means talking with our family and children about ways in which we are complicit in harm and ways in which we can heal together and be accountable.

If you have capacity, commit to monthly reparations. Redistribute wealth to organizations or individuals who have been systematically under-represented or historically denied access.

~

If you're thinking that this all sounds quite radical, you're right. I have been radicalized. And not by any particular political party, extremist coalition, or outlying social group. No. I have been radicalized by Earth, by nature herself. She found me in my most vulnerable moment, sang to me of homecoming, and awakened me to my participation in upholding harmful systems. She gave me shelter, opened my eyes to the truth of our interconnectedness, and asked me to take up arms and fight for her, for us. She transformed me. Now I am one of the converted, a warrior for eco-justice and a right-relationship evangelist.

**What life events have radicalized you? And by this I mean, what have you witnessed or experienced that cracked open your heart and spurred you to center activism in your life?**

**What are the thematic areas that you most strongly associate with your activism? For me this includes the themes of community organizing, creative guidance, and storytelling as a form of shifting cultural narratives. Make a list for yourself. Pick one and free-write or cluster map on that topic for 15 minutes. Then pick another and another. When you've finished, re-read what you've written. Did**

**writing about your activism in this way give you new insight to the ways in which you take action?**

**I mentioned earlier that my stated goal as a creative and artist is collective liberation and right-relationship. What are your goals? What dreams do you hold as central to your creative work?**

## INTEGRATION

When I first begin to write something, I include every little detail and anecdote that resonates with me. I include it all as fuel for take-off. In the beginning of any creative project, I am not a keen judge of what to keep or jettison, because I don't yet know how to fly the aircraft. Once I'm in the air, writing into the heart of my subject, all the extra sentences that helped me get off the ground become dead weight, dragging down the work and slowing my trajectory.

In her book *The Writing Life*, Annie Dillard writes, "Sometimes the writer leaves his early chapters in place from gratitude; he cannot contemplate them or read them without feeling again the blessed relief that exalted him when the words first appeared—relief that he was writing anything at all. That beginning served to get him where he was going, after all; surely the reader needs it, too, as groundwork. But no." Just like Robert's overburdened pear tree, we must trim away the extra fruit. Look at the cluster of options, identify the most promising one, and cut the rest away. Use the shears.

We can employ this method with our art, but we can also use it as a way to hone our activism. When working alongside communities most affected by supremacy systems, there is no need to recount the story of your awakening or the inciting incident that propelled you into action. That is for your own awareness and analysis. Instead, focus on radical listening and informed action. Radical listening refers to listening with intent to understand. And informed action is the capacity to take action influenced, informed and centered by the lived experience of those impacted by systemic inequity rather than on assumptions you may have about their experience. You are here in solidarity to address the immediate needs of the community. Rather than centering your past experience and creative inquiry, allow it to be the fuel that propels you into deeper relationship with those to whom you are in service.

**Where does old habit energy live in your body and in your creative work? In your activism?**

**When you look at the fruit tree of your creative life, what needs to be snipped away?**

**When you look at the systems and structures that harm you and harm others, where can you divest? Where can you step away, untangle, unhook, or even boycott?**

**In what ways have you centered yourself or your past experience in your activism?** (We've all done it.) This could look like responding to someone's story of harm or challenge with a story of your own. This could look like attempting to lead in spaces where you were not invited to lead. This could look like sharing the stories of others without permission. These look like any action you took that led you away from right-relationship.

**What is the difference for you between learning and unlearning behavior?**

**What kinds of things do you need and crave that the Earth also needs and craves?**

ONE-WORD PROMPTS FOR LITHA

Spark • Solar • Breath • Caregiver • Vision
Power • Burn • Ecosystem • Mutual Aid • Excavate
Voice • Collective • Insight • Incite • Radical
Disruptor • Chrysalis • Justice • Peace • Energy
Shears • Heal • Reciprocity • Kin • Wren
Respond • Growth • Unlock • Transform • Rest

## The Next Six Weeks

Everything offered here is simply a launch point. It's a place to begin. For those of you who are new to activism, spend some time over the next six weeks exploring where your gifts and values align. Identify what you care most about and the roles you feel most called to. How do you want to use your innate creative gifts to take action? For those of you who already activate your creative gifts for the purpose of social change, let the next six weeks be an opportunity to re-align. How have the needs of your community changed? What new skills, knowledge, or learning have surfaced as a part of your activism?

## Cross the Threshold

The fruit tree blossoms are fading. The wildflowers are spent. The Flower Moon has come and gone. And the weather reports tell me that the first real heat wave is on its way. But the show isn't over yet. Those beautiful blossoms did their job. The pollinators visited each open-hearted flower and the fruits we dreamed of in deep winter are now swelling in the growing warmth. The precious vulnerable seeds of early March are making good on their promise. So let's take their lead and also make good on the promises we made. To the earth. To each other. To our communities. And to ourselves. This is the time to deliver.

~

Sympathetic resonance is an amazing and elegant phenomenon. A musical note played out in the open will send vibrations that bring to life any resonating object of a matching tone. Everything has an energetic frequency and humans both emit and receive these vibrations. Remember the wren? You and what you are seeking have a harmonic likeness. But if you don't give voice to your dream and broadcast your song, how can it find you? Pluck the strings of your deepest desires and then listen for the sympathetic reverberations. The community you long for, longs for you. But you can't find each other unless you speak your hopes for the future aloud.

If you have a chance, light a little bonfire outside when the sun is setting. (A little indoor candle or smudge pot will work just as well.) Grab a small piece of paper and write down something you'd like to release or let go of as you welcome summer. Hold it in your hands.

Thank it for its gift and tell it that you no longer need it. Then toss it in the fire or light it with your candle and place it in a fire-safe bowl. As it transforms into ashes and smoke, give gratitude for making space for something new.

I've lit a fire too. And your fire and mine will burn together, touching the dream, as we recommit each day to our collective work for justice and right-relationship. *Piu, Piu, Piu.* The Canyon Wren is in the streets singing his song. Listen, do you hear it? Let's join him.

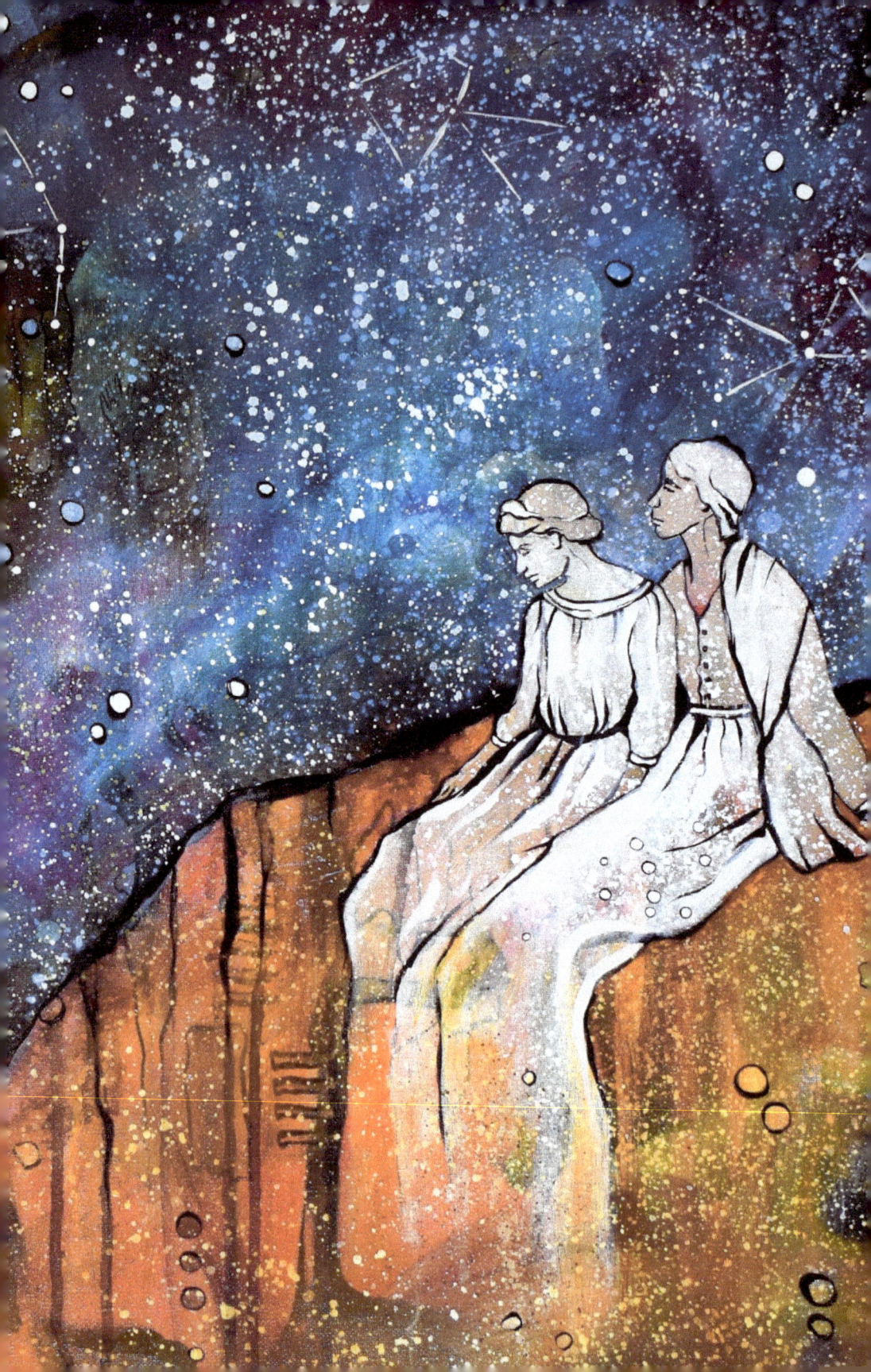

# 6

# WE ARE SKY: LUGHNASA

## ACCOUNTABILITY PRACTICE

**The Call:** Reciprocity is sacred.

**The Question:** How does my creative practice nurture right-relationship?

**The Time:** August 1 and 2

**The Origin:** Lughnasa (pronounced LOO-na-sah) is the first harvest festival on the Celtic calendar and marks the halfway point between the summer solstice and the autumn equinox. Traditional Lughnasa festivals are a time of feasting, trading, and community conversation and negotiation.

**The Imagery:** Bread, Fruit, Cornucopia Basket

**The Themes:** Reciprocity, Responsibility, Accountability, Harvest

THE FIRST HARVEST OF THE SEASON HAS ARRIVED. EARTH SHOWERS US WITH riches and invites us to share the plenty, redistribute the wealth, and acknowledge all who made harvest possible. Let this season's harvest shatter the illusion of ownership. Everything we have is a gift from the living Earth. We own none of it, but are instead its stewards, siblings, and soul-friends. We are visitors here. This land does not belong to us. We belong to the land.

The poet Rumi tells us, "Let the beauty we love be what we do. There are hundreds of ways to kneel and kiss the ground." The beauty we love is Nature's creation. How we kneel and kiss the ground is up to us. What will we do to practice accountability with people, seeds, plants, minerals, rocks, waterways, soil, and all of Earth's many gifts? And what happens when we are out of alignment? How do we find our way home when we have unintentionally created harm?

This chapter is filled with creative inquiries and inspiration for building right-relationship with people, land, plants, and animals. Creativity plays an enormous role in how we form our ideas about the world and about ourselves. This is why I feel it is imperative that we marry our creative process with an accountability practice. This season, Lughnasa asks us to allow our mistakes to work their magic. But the magic won't simply happen on its own. This kind of growth requires that we tend to our mistakes, learn from them, take risks, and surrender our addiction to quantifiable outcomes.

CALLING YOU HOME – A SEASONAL HOMILY FOR LUGHNASA

"Yes, but how do we live in right-relationship?"

I was on a three-person panel for a conference at the Dallas Symphony Orchestra and we were discussing gender equity in the music business. This was a question from the audience directed at me. She cleared her throat and continued, "You mentioned right-relationship and I'm just wondering how we do that?"

I looked around at the room. It was filled with musicians, artists, and upper-level management from some of the most prestigious arts institutions in north Texas. These were people I wanted to work for. I knew they wouldn't like my answer. "If we are to live in right-relationship," I began, "we have to talk about identity, power and accountability. Who are we and are we allowed to show up whole in the workplace? Are we willing to shift power-dynamics that silence the many in service of the few? And is there a process in place for when we mess up?"

She looked around at her colleagues. "That sounds hard," she said.

In its simplest form, accountability is the state of being responsible or answerable for the impact of our actions and behavior. More broadly, it applies to being accountable for the impacts of a system and its behavior. Oppressive systems don't maintain themselves. They need people to maintain them.

My calling as an artist is to invite my community into a state of right-relationship, which means I have to weave a robust account-ability practice into my creative work. I want to create in a way that reduces suffering and even heals.

So where do we start? We start with ourselves. We start at home.

～

It was the first day of August and I was deadheading in my mother's flower garden. She would have done it herself, but after forty-plus years on her feet as a hair-dresser, arthritis had overwhelmed her hands and lower back. She couldn't squeeze the shears anymore. But she loved her flowers and I welcomed the opportunity to spend time in her garden.

I talked to the seed pods and sang little prayers of gratitude as I pruned. The hollow stems of Allium and Poppy snapped off easily, while the Hollyhock and Rudbeckia required the snippers. The wild arms of the Russian Sage were still going strong, so I left them alone. A husky, orange-bottomed bumble bee landed on one of its thin purple limbs. It bowed down in supplication under the weight. Even the Russian Sage has found a way to kneel and kiss the ground.

That day, kneeling in my mother's garden, looking around at the flowers, the farmhouse, and the hayfields beyond, I was filled with a complex sense of gratitude. I was thankful for our home, which shel-ters our dreaming and safety. I was thankful for the soil under my fingernails, the Cottonwoods along the creek, and the water that rolled through the valley and gave life to everything. But I also recognized a deeper sense of responsibility for its health and longevity. Underscoring this immense feeling of home and stewardship was the knowledge that I am a settler here. Wherever I lay my head, I am on indigenous land.

Do you know where your people are from and how it is that you've come to this moment? Do you know your history? If we are to live, work, and create in right-relationship, we must know ourselves and the legacies to which we are connected. To engage in culture-shift requires that we first understand the culture(s) that made us.

I come from Celtic people who emigrated to the US during the Clearances in Scotland and the famines in Ireland. In my matrilineal line, many of my people spent their lives working as day laborers and migrant farm hands throughout the country: Minnesota, Nebraska, Kansas, and Wyoming. They even made it to southern Canada during the Dust Bowl. In my patrilineal line, we worked as stonemasons and laundresses in the east, building the cities of Pittsburgh and Washington DC. My people may have been outsiders upon arrival, but as our young country grew into its adolescence, my immigrant ancestors were soon absorbed into a culture of whiteness that rewarded their assimilation and obeisance. And some of those rewards came in the form of access to real estate.

This farmhouse stood empty for almost five years before my mom and her late husband decided to make it their home. The house was in terrible shape and needed long-term attention and rehabilitation. I share this with you because in its current state, after decades of hard work and sweat equity, this home is its own kind of harvest for our family. We brought babies into the world here and we buried our dead here.

While this place is the culmination of our family's generational work and fortitude, our ability to buy property at all in the past three generations is largely due to bank practices that made home loans available to white soldiers and working-class families. These opportunities were specifically withheld from Black families. And if we were to spiral back even further, we'd see that this fertile valley was home to a multitude of native tribes like the Nimiipuu, Cayuse, Walla Walla, and others.

Part of my work to be in right-relationship with this land is not only to honor the sovereignty and wisdom of these people but to unlearn the devastating tools of their colonizers, from which I descend. And contextualizing the story of our home helps me to own the truth of my family's assimilation and participation in settler colonialism.

As I deepen into a reparatory relationship with this land, I continue to ask what is mine to do in healing the harm? The woman at the Dallas Symphony Orchestra was right about accountability – it's hard. But if we are to create a livable future for the generations to come, we need to reckon with our history of this land. These seven acres hold a complicated legacy. I'm humbled and grateful to be a part of its current conversation.

Lughnasa invites us to hold this year's harvest with both hands, innately worthy of its gifts, but also aware of the land's sovereignty and our responsibility as one of its stewards. Let's weave reciprocity and right-relationship into our creative practices as a form of cultural wound-tending. Come, kneel in the soil, and bow down like the sage under the weight of the bee. Mother Earth is calling us to love her back into wholeness. And in doing so, we'll heal ourselves.

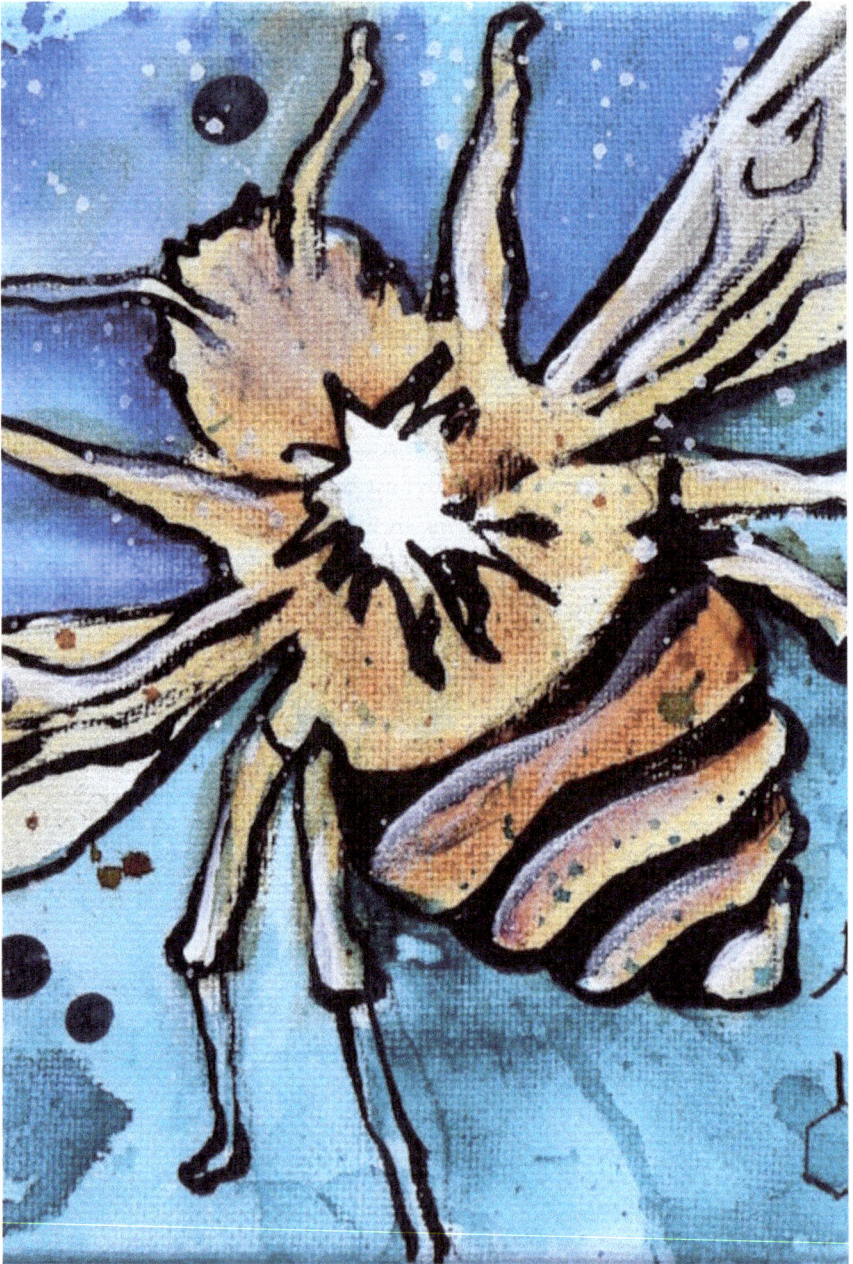

Tend the Altar

In Irish Gaelic, the word for August is *lunasa*. Lughnasa marks the halfway point between the summer solstice and the autumn equinox and it always falls on August first. This ancient Gaelic feast-day honors the Irish deity Lugh, the God of skill. He is traditionally honored with corn, grains, bread, and other symbols of the harvest. Later, in Christian England the date was called Lammas, after the Saxon phrase that translates to "loaf mass." In its most basic form, Lughnasa is a bread holiday, an Irish tribute to carbohydrates. My kind of holiday.

Food is a gift from Earth and sky and pollinators. Anytime food is available to us, it means that many people and other sentient beings were involved in its creation, fruition, harvest, preparation, and delivery. That's why food is a great place to start when talking about right-relationship.

I'm a food person. I dream food, talk food, think food, and all my memories are connected to food. Katie, my oldest child, likes to pop-quiz me about what I was eating and when. If, for instance, my partner is reminiscing aloud about a day in 2002 when we visited a friend in Monterey, Katie will interject, "Mom! Quick. What did you have for dinner that night." Everyone laughs as I detail the tapas restaurant at the edge of the bay, the calamari which arrived not fried as expected, but lightly grilled with lemon juice and capers, the freshness of the Roma tomatoes in the caprese salad, the granular texture of the Gruyère cheese on the charcuterie plate, and each wine pairing.

It was only natural that my love of food led me to gardening. I wanted to put delicious, wholesome, organic food on our family's table. I planted my first raised vegetable bed when my kids were still very little. I wanted them to enjoy the sheer pleasure of popping a warm unwashed strawberry into their mouths. I wanted them to experience the sensation of snap peas off the vine and crunched between their teeth.

This was a great plan in theory. But the reality was that my son Charlie wasn't going to be popping strawberries or crunching snap peas. He'd had a stroke and could barely even take a bottle. In those early years, life with Charlie centered around what he could and could not eat. Neurologists sent us for swallow studies, speech therapy, eating classes, and x-rays of his esophagus, which exposed muscular slack and aspiration. It quickly became clear that Charlie would not be transitioning to solid food. Maybe, ever.

Would Charlie ever experience the silliness of pitting a cherry with his teeth, or joyfully slurp up homemade pasta, or tongue peanut butter off the roof of his mouth, or know the exquisite pleasure of the combination of cheesecake, raspberry coulis, and graham cracker crust? It was just another thing Charlie would never do in a long line of heart-breaking "never dos."

We made a garden nonetheless. Besides, I figured that anything grown in the dirt could also go in a blender.

I started small. My goal was to make yummy food, but I also wanted to disrupt the mainstream American cultural narrative that viewed the household as a unit of consumption. I wanted to reclaim my life and stop the cycles of grocery store spending that were happening for our young family. Plus, Charlie's medical care was chaotic and uncertain at best. A garden felt like a great way to ground my energy and focus on something lifegiving.

Now, it wasn't like I was milking goats in my backyard or installing a composting toilet or anything. I also wasn't interested in dragging my household back in time - I had studied Betty Friedan's *The Feminine Mystique* and knew my way around *Feminism is for Everybody* by bell hooks. My eyes were wide open on that score. But I was really excited to produce our own food, simplify our spending, consume less from corporations, decrease our waste, support local farmers and enrich our local community through our efforts.

The unexpected gift of eating from our own garden was how it illuminated the web of relationship between our family and everything else. It made us mindful of how we ate, what was in season, ethical harvesting practices, where our food came from, and the long chain of people and places that had a hand in its creation. Zen Buddhist Thich Nhat Hanh isn't overstating when he writes, "In this food I see clearly the presence of the entire universe supporting my existence." Tending that tiny sliver of Earth, kneeling in the dirt and gathering greens, our family woke up to the divine order of reciprocity. And we were richly rewarded. The color in Charlie's face improved because of the nutrient-dense food he was ingesting. And blood tests later confirmed what we could see with our own eyes. That same year, when Charlie began making his first clear speech sounds, our neurologist credited the boost in brain-building food as a key factor. The health of the Earth is intricately connected to the health of all living things.

ALTAR PRACTICE

Lughnasa is a loaf-mass, a bread holiday symbolized by the cornucopia basket of Earth's overflowing abundance. So let's break bread. The invitation this season is to consider our kitchen tables as a place to practice right-relationship. Think of all the things that happen at your table: early morning coffee, meals, meetings, paperwork, conversations, school studies, and more. Our communal table is an altar devoted to daily life. I can't imagine a better place to engage in acts of reciprocity and accountability than at the kitchen table.

Prepare your table as you would your altar. Speak a blessing for right-relationship as you wipe the surface. Imagine that you are clearing old habit energy and priming the space for open-hearted dialogue, honest words, compassionate action, and nourishing meals. Choose a candle for the center of the table. Before sitting down to meals or conversations, set an intention for your time and light the candle. Your intention could be as simple as "May I be mindful of my words," or "May we listen to understand." Setting a mutual intention can be especially powerful when you're sitting down for a hard conversation with someone you love. Author and facilitator adrienne maree brown also recognizes the power of the communal table and has developed a style of transformative justice that she calls "kitchen table mediation." This is where people in conflict sit down at a literal kitchen table for a facilitated conversation. The kitchen table altar is a powerful place from which to set the tone for your household and family life.

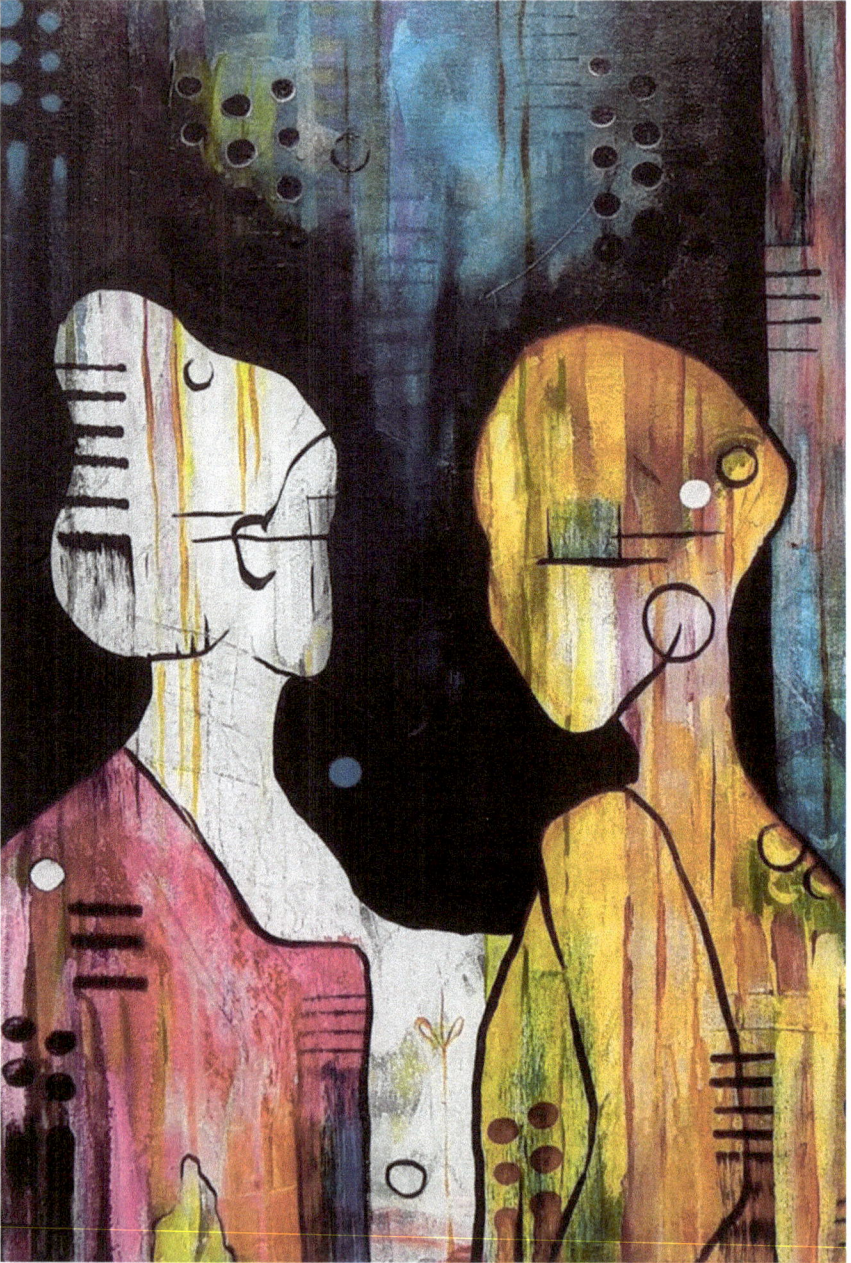

### ACCOUNTABILITY PRACTICE

The evolution of our learning and growth is built upon our capacity for adaptation and change. Mistakes are inevitable. Let's allow ourselves to learn from them. Who might we be if we embraced our mistakes as an opportunity for creative innovation, rather than something to hide or sprint past? Author and disability justice activist Mia Mingus tells us that "the only way to get skilled at accountability is to practice it and the only time we can truly practice it is when we have messed up or caused or been complicit in harm." There is magic in our mistakes, but we must have the courage to risk being wrong.

I want to name here that as a white-bodied person, practicing accountability is life-long. My colonial programming is so deep that there are times when I am not even conscious of the ways in which I show up as a colonizer. Despite my good heart, my open eyes, my ongoing education, and my anti-racist practices, I will cause harm. And the Black, Indigenous, and People of Color that I am in relationship with will witness and feel that harm. This is why I am devoting an entire chapter to an exploration of accountability and repair. When white folks are called to activist work, we must also be committed to an authentic and honest accountability practice.

A society that cannot face its past transgressions cannot heal or move forward. It is the same for individual relationships. As you read on, I encourage you to hold reciprocity and accountability as holy artforms. These prompts and stories are meant to deepen self-awareness, identify points of engagement, and empower you to use your creative gifts in service of healing.

### INCUBATION

All accountability work begins with self-awareness and self-knowledge. Exploring our identity is the first step towards building an accountability practice. For this work, let's look to the study of Bioculture, which is a combination of biological and cultural factors that affect human behavior.

If you've ever applied for a job, written a grant, or been a college student, you've likely been asked to create a resume or a short biography. These perfunctory tools usually share a bit about your education and experience and perhaps some special skills you've picked up along the way. They're also used to share why you are the right person for the job. For our purposes, I'd like to create a different kind of biography, one in which we excavate our culture and personal values rather than our industry-approved qualifications.

**Cultural Biography**

A cultural bio is a great way to begin the work of socially and culturally locating ourselves before stepping into liberatory justice work. It might seem limiting at first, but ultimately it gives us full permission to inhabit our own lineage, draw from its legacy, and engage in social justice work centered in the truth of our history. Let's spend some time creating our own cultural biography. For the moment, set aside your college degree and work history and pick up your family tree and/or lived experience.

Here are some journal questions to get you started:

**Describe your cultural identity or ethnicity. And where are the original lands of your people?**

**What family traditions did you have growing up? Were these traditions inherited from generations past? Or did you create them in the absence of generational traditions?**

**What is a unique belief held by your traditional community or cultural group?**

**Did anyone in your family history speak another language at some point? When did your family lose that language and gain a new one? Why was it lost or stolen from them?**

How does your family dress for special occasions? Or how did they traditionally dress for special occasions?

How did your family participate in traditional ceremonies or religious observances?

Did you have traditional music that originated with your people?

What types of traditional foods did you harvest and cook? And what are the traditional medicinal plants used by your community?

Did your family immigrate from their country of origin to a new place? Why did they do this? Was it by choice? Circumstance? Or was it forced? What are the details of their immigration journey?

What kind of work did your ancestors do? Were there opportunities available to them after their immigration journey?

What kind of work do your grandparents and parents do now? Is it different from their recent ancestors?

When you think about access, where do you have access in your daily life? What resources do you have access to and why? How do you leverage those resources?

What life events have impacted your family story? Natural disaster, displacement, divorce, inheritances, treaties, legislation, immigration, windfalls, economic hardships, drug use, education, mental health, abuse, religious persecution, promotion, etc.

Journaling on these questions will certainly foster some new awareness, but it is also a simple way to practice truth-telling that allows you to show up in your wholeness. Your answers will serve as a foundation on which to build your cultural bio. Weave the answers to these questions in any way that feels good for you, but if you're like me and love to see examples, here are two recent biographies that I submitted for a facilitation job. I've included a traditional biography as well as a cultural biography so you can see and feel the difference. Please note that this is a snapshot in time and I may express this differently in the future.

Traditional Bio:

*Sarah Greenman is an artist, storyteller, and facilitator who has experience as a frontline staff member, educator, outreach director, birth worker, project manager, and nonprofit operations director. Sarah holds a BA in Creative Writing with an emphasis in Gender Studies from Mills College. She is also a graduate of the Pacific Conservatory Theater. Sarah is a 2021-22 fellow with the American Leadership Forum of Oregon, a Certified Narrative4 Facilitator, and a member of the Dramatists Guild. Sarah also serves on multiple boards working as a grassroots community organizer. Sarah resides in Halfway, OR with her children Katie and Charlie.*

Cultural Bio:

*Sarah Greenman (pronouns: she/they) is an artist, storyteller, and facilitator. Her work is rooted in a core framework of justice, radical inclusion, creativity, and anti-racist praxis. Sarah embodies a liberatory eco-arts practice in service of right-relationship with land, animals, plants, and people. Sarah is a curious and strategic facilitator who weaves joy, story, connection, and purpose into all of her community building work.*

*Sarah has experience as a frontline staff member, educator, outreach director, birth worker, project manager, and nonprofit operations director. Her work as a birth and death doula is particularly powerful when applied to groups interested in crossing transformative thresholds.*

*Sarah is a white, cisgender, queer, able-bodied, woman of size. She is a descendent of settler-colonizers, migrants with Celtic ancestry who came to the United States as landless farmers fleeing famine and violence from Scotland, Ireland, and Sweden. Her people were stone masons, laundresses, and day laborers.*

*Sarah grew up in Central California with two divorced, working parents (her mother was a hairdresser, her father a high school teacher.) She does not come from intergenerational wealth but her lower-middle class family always owned their home.*

*Sarah has worked as a waitress, a bartender, a line-cook, a substitute teacher, a website designer, a nanny, and a nonprofit professional. She has always had access to some kind of paid work opportunity and has never experienced houselessness. She attended and graduated from Mills College with the help of financial aid, federal student loans, and a merit scholarship; she holds a BA in Creative Writing with an emphasis in Gender Studies. She is also a graduate of the Pacific Conservatory Theater.*

*Sarah resides in Halfway, OR on the stolen ancestral lands of the Nimiipuu, Cayuse, and Walla Walla. To align her land recognition more closely with action, Sarah redistributes a percentage of proceeds from her work to local native-led community organizations.*

Creating a cultural biography can be an iterative process that continues to develop as you grow and deepen your creative work. It's a powerful tool for liberation because of its transparency. Rooting into your cultural legacy, however pained or proud you might feel about it, informs how you show up to your work as a creative. And this kind of truth-telling fosters self-awareness, regardless of whether or not you share it with others. The self-work you do in private will echo through every part of your life. When we know on whose shoulders we stand, we can take informed action in service of repair and right-relationship. For instance, since I know I come from a legacy of settler colonialism, I self-identify as the right person to engage in land-back efforts with native tribes. Because of my understanding of racist banking practices that gave my white-presenting family access to home ownership, I am called to take action on behalf of closing the racial wealth gap. Self-knowledge leads to informed action.

## ACTION

My creative practice is a long-form exploration of the ways art can be used as a vehicle for courageous conversation, social change, and healing. In my early career, however, I had no idea about the ethical implications of working in community. I don't think I even knew what I meant when I used the word "healing." When we're not clear about why we're doing something, mistakes and harm are inevitable.

One of my first big successes as a writer was a play I wrote while in my 20s about the German filmmaker and propagandist Leni Riefenstahl. Leni was one of 113 filmmakers hired by the Third Reich as part of their propaganda ministry and she was the only woman. I was using her life story and "art" to address questions I had about artistic responsibility. I was also trying to understand the nature of collective violence and was using the Holocaust to explore how media compelled the citizenry of an entire nation to allow the annihilation of their Jewish population. During the play's first production, I did an interview with a reporter from *The Jewish Review*. I was asked if I was Jewish. No. Was I connected to Judaism at all? Loosely. How about the play – was the director Jewish? No. Designers? No. Producers? No. I'm not proud to tell you that I had never even considered my own identity when deciding if I was the right person to tell this story.

I had put my creative ideas and goals before the wellbeing of the people it most affected. I had centered my desire to tell the story instead of seeing my work as a part of a larger conversation in which the community and I were interdependent. This interview was a turning point in my creative work. It didn't matter what talents or gifts I possessed – I needed to learn what it meant to create in community. This led to a 20-year journey to learn and integrate relational, community building skills into my creative practice.

**Conscientious Creative Practice**

It doesn't matter whether we are professional artists or private creatives. It doesn't matter whether we have an audience of millions or an audience of one. Our creative practice needs to be conscientious. It's as important for our own wellbeing as it is for others because our liberation is bound together. It is interconnected, interdependent, and collective.

Here are some of the guidelines I use to nurture right-relationship in my creative practice:

- Lead with curiosity and ask lots of questions.
- Let new information change you. Be susceptible.
- Tell stories that are yours to tell. (Don't share stories that are not yours.)
- Slow down. Most harm occurs when we go fast.
- Practice apologizing. (We're terrible at it.)
- Cite your sources. This may sound small, but when it comes to creative ideation, we need to give credit where credit is due.
- Handle mistakes publicly and with transparency.
- Make clear invitations for feedback and a timely response process.
- Define your terms. Build your own glossary so that when you speak, you can do so with courage and conviction.
- Diversify your bookshelf. Read the works and theory of authors who do not look like you or have your same lived experience.
- Support Black-owned bookstores and art shops when purchasing your materials.
- Use and make environmentally sustainable art materials.
- Take responsibility for your own education. It's not the job of the oppressed to educate the oppressor.
- Participate in local truth and reconciliation efforts with your local tribes.

- Don't do it alone. Seek out accountability partners and mentors.
- Pay people of color for their work. Did you learn something from them? Pay them. Did you ask them for their time? Pay them. Do you appreciate their offer? Pay them.
- Champion other creatives and artists of color. Speak their names in rooms where you have influence.

～

**Dreaming Accountability**

When we begin to expand our accountability practice, we sometimes run into our own shame, fear, and trauma. In her article "Dreaming Accountability," Mia Mingus writes, "What if accountability wasn't scary? It will never be easy or comfortable, but what if it wasn't scary? What if our own accountability wasn't something we ran from, but something we ran towards and desired, appreciated, held as sacred? What if we cherished opportunities to take accountability as precious opportunities to practice liberation? To practice love?"

Let's grab our journals and use Mia's question as inspiration to address some of the feelings that may be coming up for us:

**What if accountability wasn't scary? What if our own accountability wasn't something we ran from, but something we ran towards and desired, appreciated, held as sacred?**

**What if we cherished opportunities to take accountability as precious opportunities to practice liberation? To practice love?**

And some of my own questions:

**When in your life have you caused harm but felt afraid to repair? What caused this fear? How did your harm perpetuate and maintain a culture of harm? And how would you like to be accountable in the wake of that harm now?**

**How does accountability inform our own creativity? Or flip it: how does creativity inform our own accountability?**

～

## Honor the Land

Just as we honor people, we can honor the land on which we stand. My own art studio is situated on the traditional and unceded lands of the Nimiipuu, known federally as the Nez Perce. This simple fact compels me to explore ways in which I can heal my fractured relationship with the land and the descendants of her original people. We cannot engage with the land and remain separate from it.

Before we discuss honoring land and reparations, I want to name once again that I am a student and practitioner of this work and not a source of theory, history, or leadership. Leadership comes from your local tribes and community centers for social change and movement building. There is no blueprint for how to engage in land reparations. Every region and tribe is different in its history and experience of colonization.

This book shares a permission-giving process that asks you to take creative risks, to explore and experiment. That's why I encourage you to find creative ways to weave in reparations and honoring land as you gather friends, create work, run your business, and show up in community. Thoughts and practices that honor land are ever-evolving. Everyone on this planet is in an iterative learning process as we move further towards right-relationship. Inform yourself by connecting with respect and deference to your local tribal organizations. I don't mean to say that we show up on the doorsteps of local tribal centers and say, "Hey, I'm here to help." No. This is an invitation to engage in culturally appropriate ways: donate funds, research and participate in land-back efforts, follow your local tribal social media and answer their public announcements for community volunteer opportunities. Deep listening is paramount as we build capacity for accountability and repair.

I began my journey with a full year of monthly donations to a local

Nimiipuu Organization. I received a letter of thanks from one of their board members and was able to respond by offering my time. A few months later, I received a call from their volunteer coordinator asking if I'd be interested in participating in a work party to restore a barn on some newly acquired property. Go slow. Be intentional. And center their voices, stories, needs, and requests. And remember that right-relationship is a practice, not a destination.

It is an honor to be in relationship with local indigenous communities. Building a meaningful relationship takes time. Centering tribal leadership, deep listening, and authentic presence is the only way I know to do this work. My goal is to be an effective and committed partner for reconciliation and reparation efforts. Here are some other ways to build your own accountability practice that honors land:

**Offer public recognition and respect to local tribes and land on which you live and work. You can do this when gathering with friends and colleagues. You can also do this on your public website or blog if you have one. Many contemporary land acknowledgments unintentionally perpetuate false ideas about the history of dispossession and the current realities for Indigenous people. Take your cues from tribal leaders. It's also important that your land acknowledgement does not exist in a past tense. Colonialism is happening now. And keep in mind that land acknowledgments are toothless and performative if you do not also take action to support tribal sovereignty and engage in reparations.**

**Support larger truth-telling and reconciliation efforts in your community by seeking out other organizations already engaged in this work. Look to see if there are Indigenous folks on the board.**

**If you are able, make monthly donations to tribal-led organizations. I feel that a small monthly donation is better than a larger one-time sum. This encourages long-form relationship building. Make sure you sign up for their newsletter and respond to any calls for support or volunteer opportunities.**

~

Here are some questions to explore in your journal or sketchbook:

How might you weave honoring land and reparations into your work and family life?

Do you know where your water comes from? Map your local watershed in your sketchbook.

What are some of the other land-based resources you make use of in your everyday living? Consider the materials used to build your home or apartment, clothes in your closet, food in your pantry, supplies in your home office, electricity grid, fuel for automobiles, etc. How are they connected to native land?

What does "colonizer" mean to you?

How does colonization show up in your thoughts, habits, relationships, education, parenting, creative practice, workspace, community, and country? This can be both as colonizer and colonized.

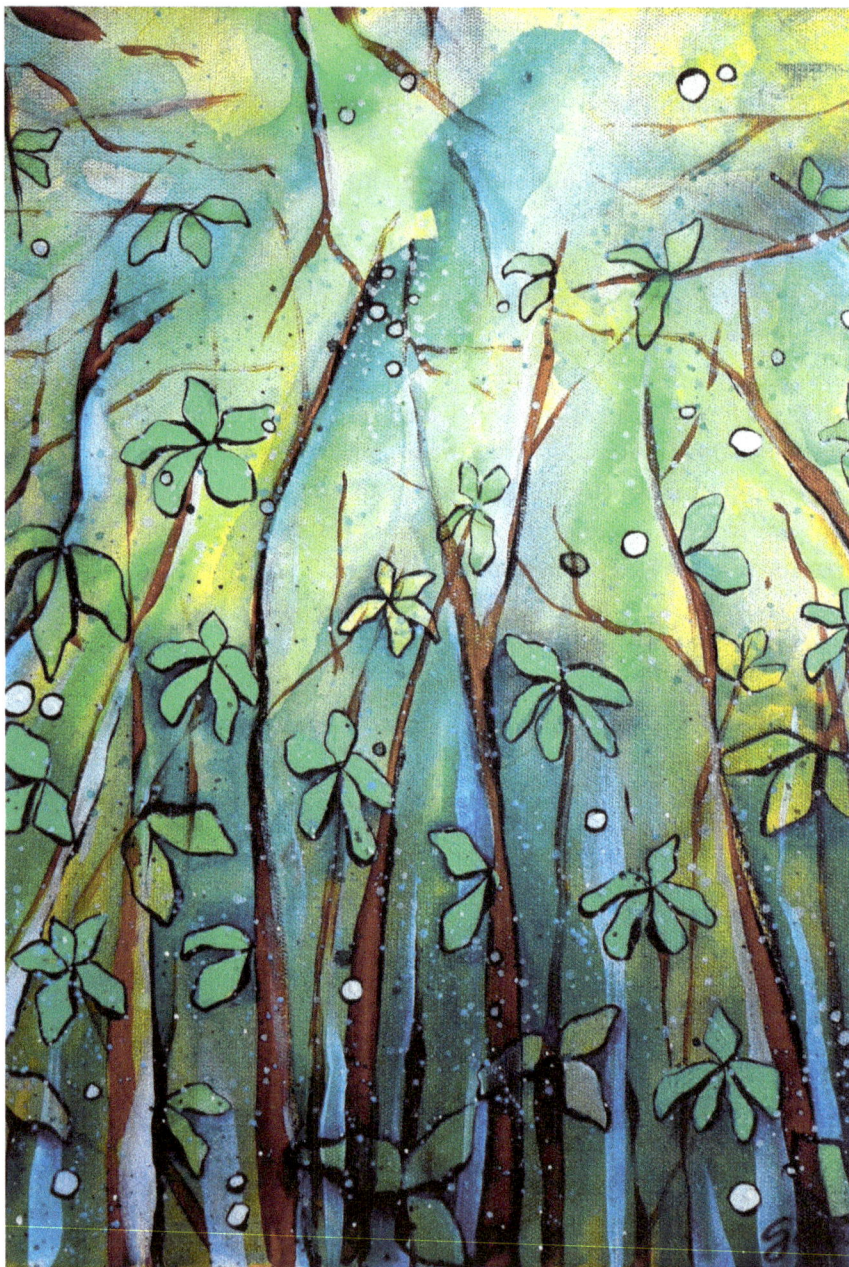

Mother Earth is a creator. Just like us. And she deserves our time and energy. Rowen White is a seed keeper, activist, and farmer from the Mohawk community of Akwesasne. She introduced me to a profound idea about reciprocity with seeds: that anytime we eat, it is because seeds and plants have kept their time-honored promise to hold and nourish us. The question Rowen poses concerns *our* promise to nourish the seeds and plants. I want us to expand our accountability practice to include not only people, but also seeds, plants, minerals, rocks, waterways, soil, and all of Earth's gifts.

## Plant Allies

Lughnasa is the first harvest festival on the Wheel of the Year. For pastoralists like the Celtic people, this time of year marked the fruition of both cultivated and wild plants. There are a variety of wild plants that were sacred to the Celts, including Foxglove, Chamomile, Dandelion Root, Hawthorne, Willow, and Passiflora. I no longer reside on the land of my ancestors, but instead live in the high desert of Eastern Oregon. My creative journey has led me to develop lasting botanical relationships with this relatively new-to-me landscape. This entails honoring old covenants with new friends.

At this time of year, I spend time in the mountains communing with one of my favorite plants, *Artemisia tridentata,* also known as sagebrush. This plant has surrounded me for most of my life in the western United States. Developing a relationship with sagebrush is one of the tangible ways I explore right-relationship with land and what it means to belong to each other. *Artemisia tridentata* thrives here in Baker County and over the past few years, after some deep listening and respectful conversations, we've become close friends.

When I harvest this plant I follow a few self-imposed rules. I always kneel beside it and ask for permission. Then I listen deeply for its reply. This information comes to me in a somatic way, a kind of language translated by skin and air. If we're in agreement, I speak aloud my gratitude and harvest a bit. Also, I never take more than half of the plant. Most herbs, cultivated as well as wild, respond well to a healthy trim, but full removal is devastating to the wellbeing and longevity of the plant. I also like to sketch the plant I harvest into my sketchbook as a kind of visual prayer. Here are some questions for your journal and sketchbook practice:

**Are there native plants in your area that you've grown close to or built a relationship with?**

**Which plants soothe you? Call to you? Teach you? Listen to you? Heal you? Confuse you? Excite you?**

**Are there any plants that nourish a sense of belonging for you? Your family? Your home?**

～

### Enough-ness

I'd like to explore this idea further. Lughnasa asks us to think deeply about the meaning of the word "harvest". There are limitless ways to share the bounty and attend to the needs of our communities. Harvest is not simply about what we individually might store away in the cellar, it's about resources we might collectively reap and distribute. Abundance is real. There is enough for all, so long as we are in right-relationship with our sense of enough-ness. Tarana Burke, the founder of the Me Too movement writes, "If I found a healing tree in my back-yard, and it grew some sort of fruit that was a healing balm for people to repair what was damaged, I'm not going to just harvest all of those fruits and say, 'You can't have this.' If I have a cure for people, I'm going to share it."

**Do you know what "enough" feels like for you and your family?**

**And how might you redistribute some of your resources as a means of creating community, connection, and a sense of communal security and belonging?**

**Do you know when you are truly and appropriately fed, clothed, comforted, sheltered, educated, held, safe, secure, and resourced? Or do you always feel that there must be more in the cellar, more in the account, more in the lock box? Can you feel when the balance tips and you are over-resourced? Over-fed? Over-housed? Over-comforted?**

**Are you afraid to let go of your overage? And do you practice re-distribution? I'm not talking about a rainy-day fund or an insurance policy on your home. I'm not talking about romanticizing deprivation. I'm talking about extra. I'm talking about consuming more than you truly need for a healthy sense of 'enough'. How might you redistribute what you do not need?**

**And what if the family next door requires more or less to reach their own understanding of enough? What if they care for a child with intersecting disabilities or medical needs. Their sense of 'enough' will likely look different from yours. What if another family tends farmland or travels for work or lives intergenerationally? Their sense of enough will probably look different than yours. Are you able to understand your own unique sense of enough-ness in the face of difference?**

**And what is your relationship with what you feel you are 'owed' or have 'earned'?**

These are the questions we need to ask ourselves as we look our time squarely in the eye and consider how to best nurture mutual care and reciprocity in our communities.

When I settle my mind and breathe into the belly of my truth, these are the words I hear: There is no need to sell the world back to itself. There is enough for all. Let's continue to tune our ears toward the commons and away from commodities. And let's continue to ask: How can we be in robust right-relationship and root into our own understanding of enough-ness?

## ONE-WORD PROMPTS FOR LUGHNASA

Harvest • Culture • Fruition • Air • Arrive
Yield • Peach • Return • Shade • Reap
Sunburn • Dog Days • Wind • Plenty • Origin
Accountable • Lavender • Lungs • Smoke • More
Offspring • Weeds • Sky • Preserve • Drought
Legacy • Dirt • Abundance • Cloud • Freedom

## THE NEXT SIX WEEKS

As we reap this season's harvest and break bread with our kin, remember that we are not alone in this work. There are millions of others practicing right-relationship right alongside us. Big, systemic change happens in small, everyday moments. Author adrienne maree brown calls it fractal responsibility. Abandon knowing it all. Abandon the expert, the authority, the hero. Instead, let's embrace the seeking, the questions, and the collective. There are roughly six weeks between now and the autumn equinox. We covered a lot of ground in this chapter. Let's use the time before us to sit with the questions. Go slow. And do as John O'Donohue advises: "be excessively gentle with yourself."

## CROSS THE THRESHOLD

To know ourselves, to acknowledge our history, and to focus our creativity towards reciprocity and accountability is holy work. We are all imperfect vessels for this work, but we must answer Earth's call: to step further into right-relationship with everything and everyone around us. It's all part of the messy, potent, fumbling, ecstatic dance of life. And harvest season is the perfect moment along the Wheel of the Year to gather each other up, link arms, and sing aloud our communal covenants to land, seeds, trees, water, air, and sky.

Autumn is on its way. Soon the bright gold and green cornucopia of August's end will give way to wind and dust and dark. What has been given will be taken away. And when the shadows appear, we will rest well knowing that we are people who repair what we break, share what we harvest, and hold what needs healing.

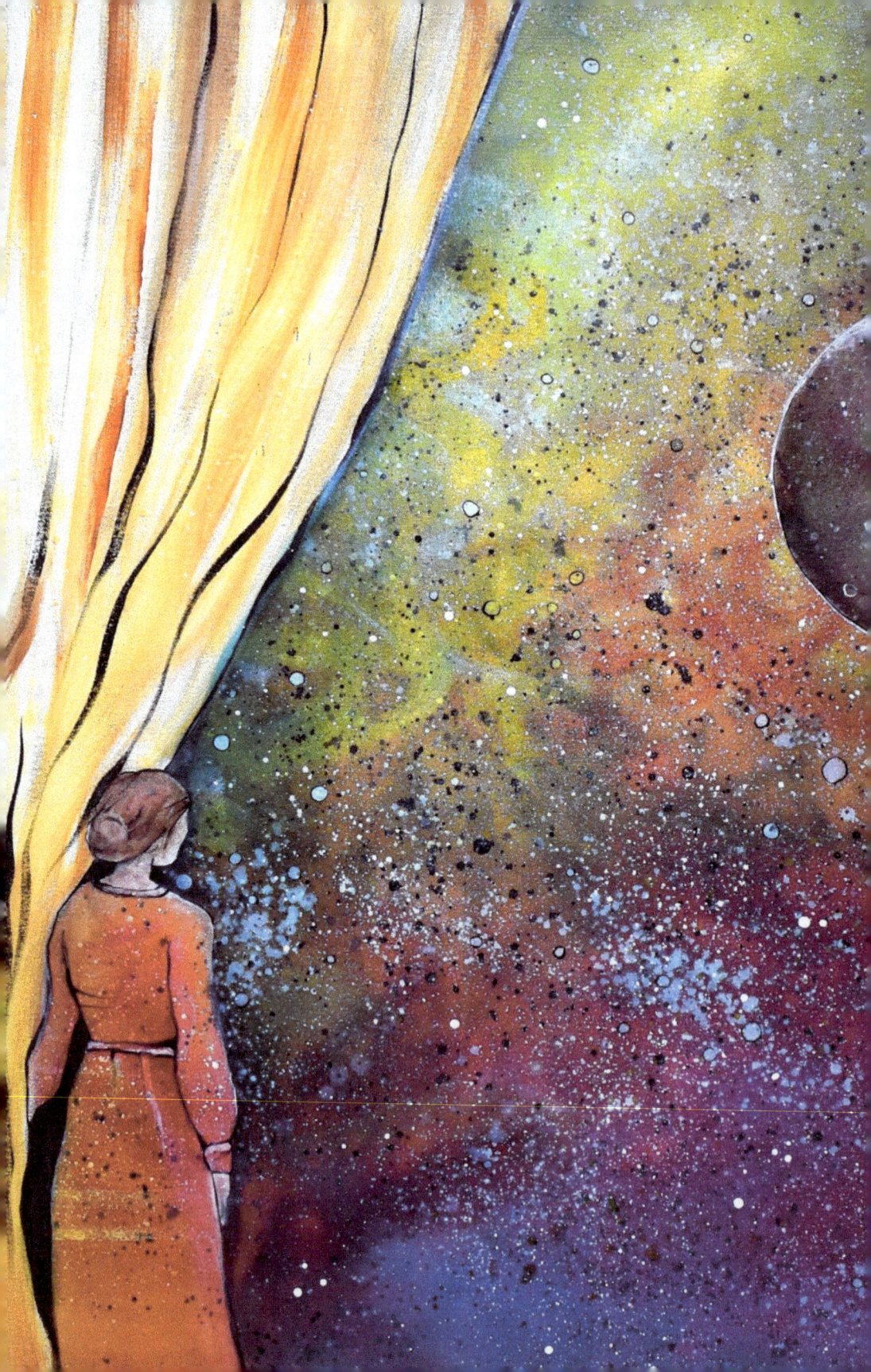

# 7

# WE ARE SEEDS: MABON

## GRATITUDE PRACTICE

**The Call:** Gratitude is the gateway to growth.

**The Question:** How can we create something new from what we already have?

**The Time:** September 19-21

**The Origin:** Mabon (pronounced MAY-bon) is a fairly new term for an ancient holiday on the Celtic calendar that marks the autumn equinox, the first day of fall, when the length of day and night are the same. In Celtic culture it marks the second harvest and is considered a thanksgiving holiday.

**The Imagery:** Seeds, Apple, Pomegranate, Harvest

**The Themes:** Gratitude, Reflection, Decay, Regeneration

ALL LIFE IS TEETERING IN THE BALANCE. THIS IS A MOMENT TO TAKE STOCK of what we have, give gratitude, and plan for the coming dark. The autumn equinox marks a moment of solar harmony as the sun moves north across the celestial equator and we embark on the dark half of the year. A Celtic thanksgiving holiday, Mabon honors the second harvest of the year. During the next six weeks, we'll celebrate this transition by weaving a gratitude practice into the very fabric of our creative work.

Over the past few decades, the self-help industry has co-opted and commodified gratitude as a practice. Gratitude is sold to us in the form of 'health and wellness," something to be cultivated as a means for building wealth, longevity, and even a kind of mental fitness. Gratitude has been relegated to the "to-do" list along with skin exfoliation and your morning protein smoothie. In this chapter we'll explore why and how gratitude is the foundation of joy, contentment, and creative flow. The greater your capacity for sincere appreciation, the deeper the connection to your heart, where intuition and unlimited inspiration and possibilities reside.

## Calling You Home – A Seasonal Homily for Mabon

The last harvest of the year is upon us. The August heat has transformed vibrant July flowers into crusty seed pods which now tremble in the September wind. Soon, they'll crack open and fulfill their true purpose, spilling their tiny seeds onto the soil below. I can hear the ache of summer's end in the sound of cawing Magpies. Today, I'm in the garden stripping tomato plants. Up here in the mountains, September is likely to catch me with a surprise overnight freeze. The first cold front of the season is sweeping down the north side of the Eagle Cap Wilderness, causing sudden gusts and dust devils along the dirt roads. The wind-chimes hanging outside my studio no longer offer sweet bell tones, but are now clacking with alarm against the eves. Mother Earth is on the move.

The first ripples of autumn's quiet transition are reaching the shores of my senses. The trees are always the first to spread the news of Persephone's descent. They call back their life force, first from their leaves and limbs, and then into their protective core, preparing for the coming cold. Trees are practiced mourners, adept at letting go. We humans should take note.

In Greek mythology, Persephone was the daughter of Demeter, Earth Goddess and protectress of all growing things. The story goes that Hades, lord of the underworld, saw Persephone in a verdant meadow gathering flowers. He, like many entitled Greek Gods, took what he wanted without asking. The ground beneath Persephone's feet opened wide and Hades dragged her down into the underworld to make her his queen.

When Demeter discovered that Persephone was gone, she fell into a state of abject grief. In her depression and sadness, Demeter neglected her duties and a great winter fell upon the Earth. Zeus, King of the Gods, asked Hades to return Demeter's daughter in order that the Earth might thrive once again. But while Persephone was with Hades, she ate the seeds of a pomegranate and in doing so, bound herself in marriage to Hades and awakened her understanding of the soul's eternal nature and the wisdom of death and regeneration. (I've noticed we humans love the recurring theme of women awakening their innate knowledge by eating orchard fruits.)

So Zeus struck a bargain with Hades for Persephone to return to her mother for half of the year. This myth feels like the first-ever joint custody agreement. Persephone returns to her mother every spring and on the autumn equinox, makes the journey back to her husband, Hades, and rules as queen of the dead. Persephone is a figure that holds both the mystery of life giver and the power which withdraws life.

My own relationship with Persephone is most prominent at this time of year. She is a beautiful representation of the "shadow self". No one is as capable of gratitude as one who has known loss and emerged from the darkness. Her annual return to the underworld is an affirmation for me that to live a fully integrated creative life, we must acknowledge our rage, our grief, and our darker emotional cosmology. Persephone is a deity that embodies creative solitude, reflective silence, and gratitude as a pathway for gestational growth.

~

Rob and Linda Cordtz own and operate an organic orchard and for the last few summers, I've worked on their thinning and harvest crew. They'd balk at my use of the words "own and operate". They consider themselves stewards, ushers, soil-tenders.

When they first took possession of the orchard, it was in a state of half-choked death. The previous farmer had used petroleum-based fertilizers. But as Rob will tell you, the soil is the heart of the orchard. All nutrients that trees need come from the soil. These nutrients are made available by microbes in the soil. For those of you who geek out on plant biology, you'll love that these microbes use organic matter and minerals in the soil as their sustenance and their byproducts are what all plants consume as "food".

Everything that happens above ground is a result of what happens underground. And every single thing that Rob and Linda do in the orchard is designed to support this process. In this way, I suppose Rob and Linda are not tree-people, but rather soil-people. The fruit they produce is hands down the most delicious thing I've ever put in my mouth.

Many years ago, perhaps in anticipation of Persephone's return, Demeter produced a long string of warm February days that caused Rob and Linda's trees to flower out of season. When a punishing freeze came on hard in March, they lost their peach and apricot crops as well as most of their other crops. Their son responded by crowd-funding a propane heating system for their orchard to ensure that future crops wouldn't meet the same fate. Our family sent a donation and in return, Linda dedicated two trees in the orchard in honor of my children.

It was late September when I brought my boys to the orchard to choose their trees. Katie was six and Charlie was three. Linda made little tin tags with their names etched into the surface and asked them to wander the orchard and choose a tree. Katie skipped off into the cherry trees to listen, as children do with trees, for one to call their name. I followed with Charlie on my hip.

Charlie moves through life with a variety of disabilities. Approximately twelve hours after he was born, Charlie began having seizures. An MRI revealed he had suffered two strokes affecting the right side of his brain, creating severe hemiplegia in his body. Hemiplegia is when half of the body is in a state of semi-paralysis and for Charlie this manifests as Cerebral Palsy. Charlie also has another condition called Craniosynostosis. This is when two skull plates fuse prematurely in the womb, trapping the child's rapidly growing brain inside a bone encasement. Asking Charlie to choose a tree in an orchard of 1500 trees is more of a gesture, rather than an actuality. However, in our family, we assume cognition, which means that Charlie gets to participate as fully as he is able.

So off we went, Charlie in arms and Katie scurrying ahead. Katie quickly located a thriving Rainier Cherry tree, claimed it as her own, and wrapped the tin tag around a low hanging branch, like a charm bracelet around its wrist. Charlie laid his head on my shoulder and was nodding off, listening to the sound of the breeze through the trees. Katie pranced off towards the house to chase some chickens while Linda and I strolled through the orchard in hopes of locating Charlie's tree.

We found ourselves among the apricots. Charlie pulled his head off my shoulder and began to look around. Perhaps he heard something rustle in the trees or smelled the crushed clover underfoot. Perhaps he was uncomfortable or felt like switching shoulders. His head swiveled around with an awkward rolling motion, not uncommon for kids with Cerebral Palsy. I walked up the row a bit. I was startled when Charlie locked his gaze on a small, stumpy tree and grunted, gesturing to the tree before us. Linda began to laugh and said, "It looks like Charlie has chosen his tree."

I could see that Charlie's tree was unwell. Its trunk was split down the center with large patches of exposed cambium where the bark was stripped away. The base of the tree had a hole in the center of the trunk so large I could slide my hand all the way through. While the surrounding apricot trees were still covered with leaves, this tree was almost bare except for a tiny but healthy bit of foliage bunched together in its upper right hand side. The sun poured down through the open space in the orchard's canopy like a spotlight on its charred limbs. "What happened here?" I asked.

"Lightning strike", answered Rob who walked towards us as Linda tied Charlie's tin tag to a gnarly corner of the twisted trunk. "I thought the tree was dead at first, but every spring it's the first tree in the orchard to eek out an armful of apricots."

Linda leaned in. "Half of the tree *is* dead," she said, "which creates an open window of sunlight for the other half of the tree. See?" Linda pointed to the bundle of leaves on the right. "These limbs get the most sun of any in the orchard, which means it's the first to bear fruit. And because it's early in the season, we can catch a higher price for these apricots at market. Isn't mother nature creative? Sometimes the wound produces the cure."

I had grieved Charlie's birth. It's hard to admit that, but I did. I grieved for the child I had imagined. The walking, talking, swimming, dancing, singing child of my dreams. But in this moment, standing in front of this glorious hemiplegic tree, I felt the power and mystery of the underworld. This tree, like Charlie, is rooted in the most nourishing soil imaginable. It is fed, loved, and tended by the most compassionate of stewards. Above ground, it manifests as "damaged", "broken", and "disposable". But below, this stunning survivor knows how to nourish itself. Gratitude flooded the corridors of my body. What I thought was broken, was in fact whole. What I understood as lacking, was instead evidence of abundance.

Persephone reminds me to pay attention to what lies beneath. She reminds me that grief is a kind of unfolding that peels away artifice and reveals the truth of our existence. I often think of her eating those pomegranate seeds, an act that seals her connection to death and also liberates her attachment to life. Maybe that's what it means to grow up.

This year, as Persephone makes her descent and again faces the dark unknown, I want to honor those places in myself where the bark has been burned away and the wind whips through the hole in my heart. I want to look this moment squarely in the eye, wake up to the beauty of impermanence, and give gratitude for the gift of grief. Valerie Castile, the grieving mother of Philando Castile, says, "Sometimes the heart has to break for the truth to fall in."

The autumn equinox asks that we welcome both the heartbreak and the healing, the grief and the gratitude. Take stock, friends. Pack only what you need for the journey ahead. May we all crack open, spill our seeds and trust the September winds to carry us softly into the dark.

When we return, there might be apricots.

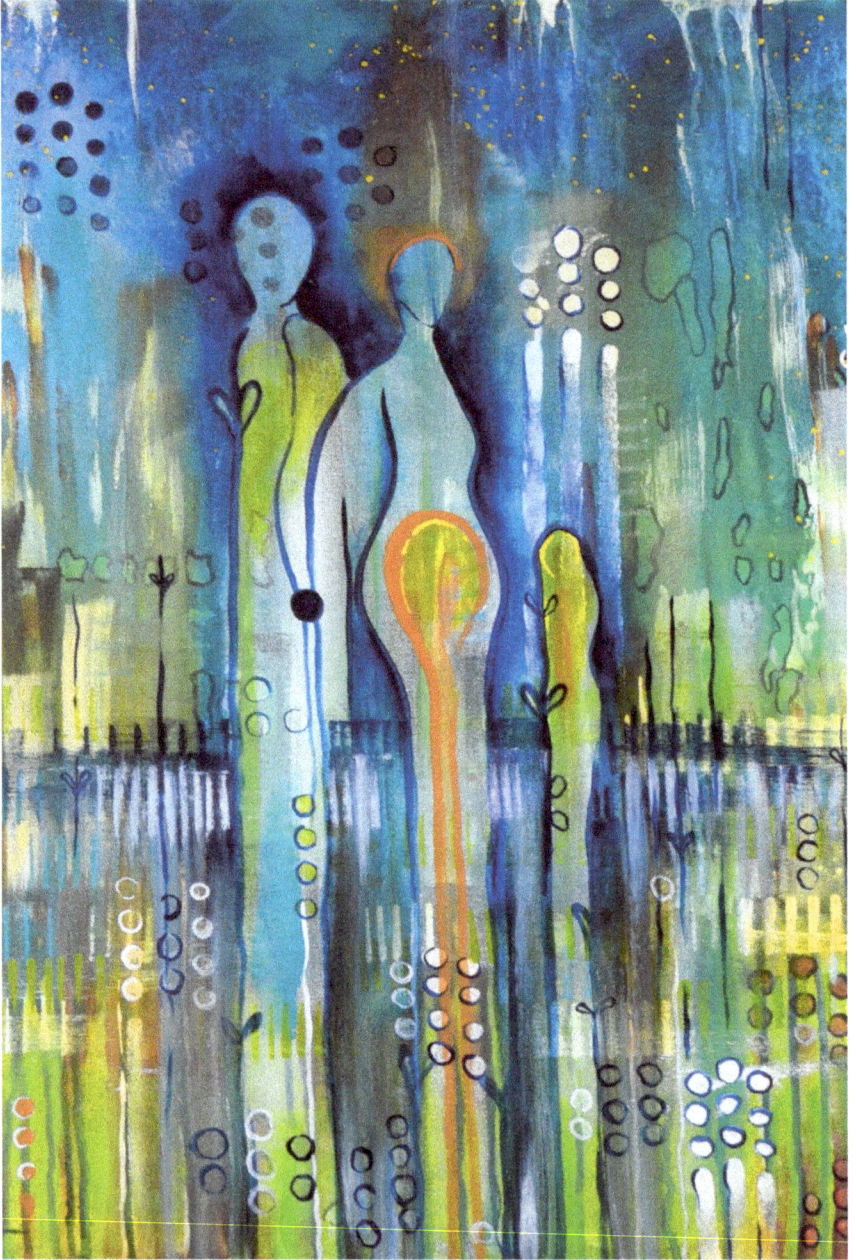

## Tend the Altar

The muse arrived today in the form of a stalk of Queen Anne's Lace, dried and dead and ready to reseed herself. Is there anything more full of possibility than a bundle of seeds? Seeds are one of the ways in which the Earth gives gratitude, both a gesture of remembrance and expansion. There is a chill in the air this morning, a kind of anticipatory breeze. It's not cold, mind you, but there is a feeling that a sharper, more exacting season is hiding just out of sight. Every living thing is once again in a state of transition. Delicious, precious transition.

## Altar Practice

Today I'm harvesting food from my friend's garden. Cassie has a fenced vegetable garden, an eighth of an acre near a small creek, perfectly situated for maximum sunlight. Since my own yard is so inhospitable to vegetable gardening with its acidic pine needles and towering conifers, I co-garden with her family each year and we share in the harvest.

But this summer, with its heat and wind and traveling for work, family obligations, and... (well... you get the idea), I have not been very present. In fact, I've been absent. I was not here to water and weed. Only twice have I visited with gloves and an hour to thin and weed, not nearly enough time to be considered a co-gardener. I was not here to sing squash and snap pea songs and sprinkle offerings onto the soil in gratitude. Others did that work. Others sang the songs and others sprinkled offerings of gratitude.

This morning, I finally had a moment to reconnect with the garden. Cassie appeared in the doorway of her house wearing a wide-brimmed hat and a handmade apron with deep pockets. I noticed beet juice stains on her front bib. Daughter Zizi followed and we all headed to the garden gate. I began to make apologies and share my reasons for being so long absent. Cassie hushed me, "There's no need to explain." She flashed a deep, knowing smile and said the temperature was expected to drop below freezing tonight. So we set our hands to work, stripping the tomato plants. The ripe ones went into our baskets for immediate use and the green ones disappeared into brown grocery bags. They need to sit on pantry shelves for a week or so to ripen.

Next we attended to the basil. Those sun loving plants would surely wilt and blacken beyond use if we left them to face the first frost. Zizi enfolded each plant in her arms, gathering all the stems together into a big hug while Cassie used a knife to cut the plant at the base. Some of the plants were hauled back to the pantry and strung upside down to dry and others would be washed and sent to the blender with garlic, olive oil, walnuts, salt, and parmesan cheese for pesto sauce.

Before I left, Cassie ducked into her pantry and emerged with gifts of chard and chiles and squash and beets and eggs — all manner of nourishment for the soul. "No," I said," this is too much. I haven't done my part." But Cassie tucked it into my arms and said "We've all done what we can and that is always enough." Gracious hosts. Gracious garden. There was enough for everyone.

～

It does not matter the reason: perhaps you've strayed or shifted priorities. Perhaps you've needed rest and time away. Consistency is not available to everyone. Life coach and author Shirin Eskandani writes, "There is an inherent privilege to 'showing up' consistently. Consistency will waver and wane as your life wavers and wanes. Be present in the season of your life, whatever that is." There is no shame in disappearing for a bit. When you feel ready, you can return, pick up your harvest basket (it's right where you left it) and step into the garden. The Earth will be waiting to welcome you home.

Mabon is one of my favorite holidays on the Wheel of the Year because it honors the light and the shadow, the waning harvest and the coming dark. Liminal space is my favorite place to dwell and make magic. Before it was called Mabon, the Celtic people called it *Meán Fómhair*, which is Welsh for Middle Harvest.

Mabon is a time for rematriation and centering the mother as the

134

source of all life. The first time I came across the word rematriation was from Martin Prechtel in *The Unlikely Peace at Cuchumaquic: The Parallel Lives of People as Plants: Keeping the Seeds Alive*. He writes that rematriation "describes an instance where land, air, water, animals, plants, ideas and ways of doing things and living are purposefully returned to their original natural context – their mother, the great Female Holy Wild." He goes on to say that rematriation is the "beginning of cultural sanity and healing."

There are so many ways to honor the great mother. All goodness begins with and returns to the land – the mother, the great Female Holy Wild. When I put my ear to the ground and listen to Earth's ever-present message, she says "remember yourself home." Remember as an active verb. Remember yourself home... to me... your mother... Danu, Gaia, Demeter, to your original context. Thank her for your life. Today, let's reseed ourselves and mark this transformational season with acts of love, reciprocity, healing, rematriation, and gratitude.

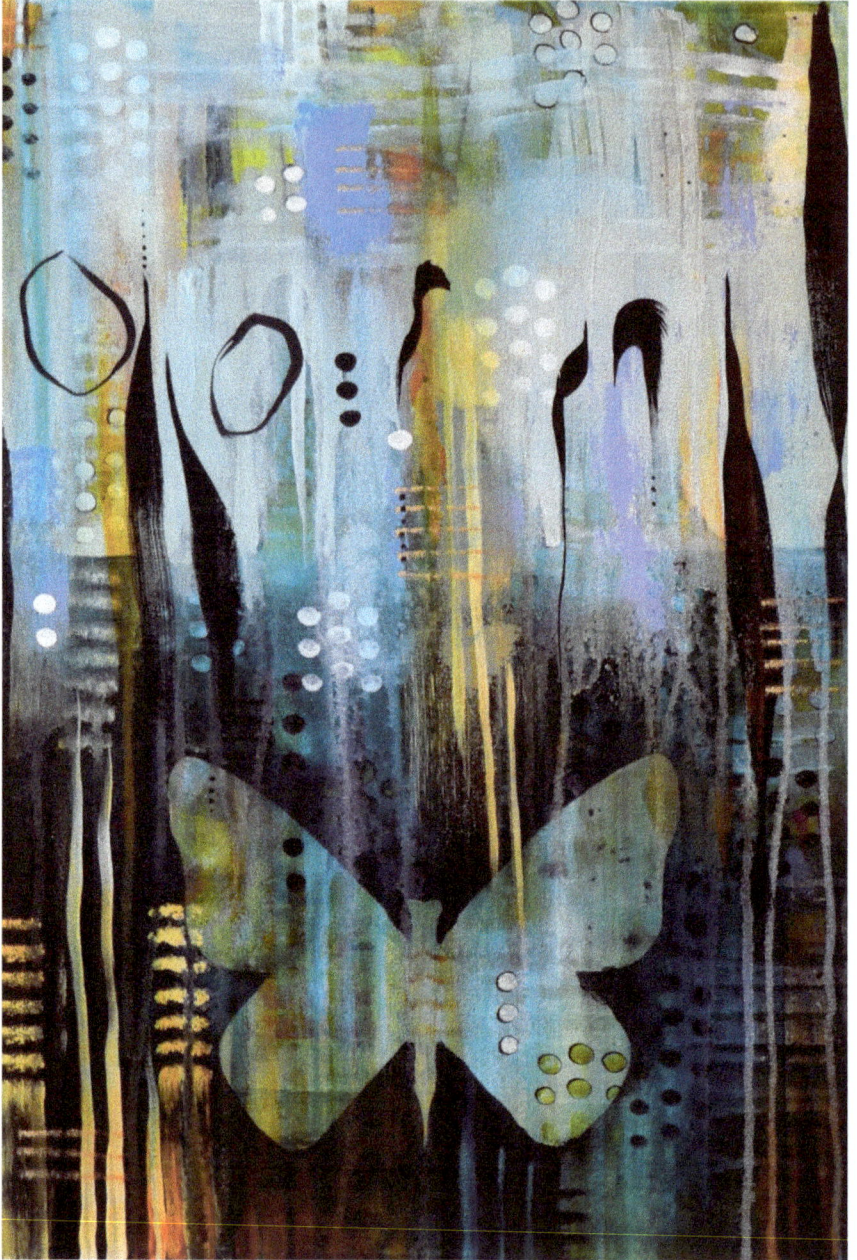

## GRATITUDE PRACTICE

I propose that gratitude is as essential as breath. Any Buddhist will tell you that it is through gratitude that we can access presence. Gratitude is a way to honor your aliveness and be a conduit for reciprocity. But gratitude isn't just something you experience alone. I believe the Earth experiences gratitude for you as well. This may seem like a big leap, but when we consider what we have been given, how can it be otherwise?

Consider that you, as you are right now, are worthy of love and liberty. Breath, nourishment, belonging, and joy are yours to have and to hold. You do not need to do anything to deserve them. They are a right. They are the manifestation of Earth's gratitude for your presence here. Just the simple fact of your being is cause for thanksgiving.

This deep knowing, that you are worthy of love and liberty, is sometimes obscured from us. Shame, isolation, trauma, or indifference can separate us from our birthright and make us feel that we are somehow separate or "other." This is why a gratitude practice is not something to check off our to-do list. It is a simple and beautiful way to support us in coming home to our true nature. Gratitude transmutes difficult moments into opportunities to practice resilience, generosity, and ease. Gratitude as remembering. Gratitude as homecoming. Gratitude as re-seeding. Gratitude as rematriation.

## INCUBATION

One of the things I'm most grateful for as a creative, is the opportunity to work in community with other makers, artists, writers, and thought leaders. The creative cross pollination that occurs in groups can be a source of potent growth and expansion. Rowen White's work and writing has had a profound effect on my creative life. Rowen has taught me not just about the rematriation of seeds but also about a "rematriation of knowledge," which rejects dominant cultural narratives and honors a return to sacred matrilineal wisdom. Rowen writes, "As a farmer and traditional seedkeeper... I can only pray that my memory and my ancestral legacy will be as that of a seedsong that is sung from the mouths of my grandchildren who know no hunger."

**What in your lineage needs healing?**

**What kind of ancestor do you wish to be?**

**Which gratitudes do you need to embody to bring about the kind of future you envision?**

**How might you share your creative work as a seedsong to be passed on to your children and grandchildren?**

ACTION

I have always wrestled with perfectionism. There was a time when I believed that if I could not do something perfectly, then there was no point in doing it at all. Perfectionism prevented me from beginning so many heart-centered projects. But now I'm learning to befriend my internal editor and take the leap even though I don't have all the answers. After taking many turns around the Wheel of the Year, I find that imperfection begets innovation. It provides a playground for my mind and hands to come alive and try new ways of making, doing, and being.

**When it comes to your creative life, what prevents you from beginning something new?** This can be a loose list or a collection of more cohesive thoughts. I offer this prompt simply as a way of identifying what barriers exist for our impulse to begin.

**Write a letter of gratitude to your imperfection.** How has imperfection created space for innovation? When has imperfection opened a door to a new way of thinking? What kind of learning has transpired because of imperfection?

We're closing in on the end of the growing season. There are signs of imperfection everywhere: unweeded garden beds, overwatered yellow leaves, under-pruned tree boughs, and even a large leafy tomato plant that didn't produce a single tomato. Some things flourished and others languished on the vine. The autumn equinox is a wonderful time to take stock and make notes for next year's garden. I like to inventory my creative work in the same manner as I do the garden. As you consider the many creative ideas and projects you set in motion this year, you'll notice that some bore fruit and others didn't. Here are some questions to take to your journal pages:

**Which creative fruits from the past season have produced viable seeds for the future?** These are efforts that nourished you and are aligned with the kind of garden you want to grow next season.

**And which of my creative fruits from the past season need to be composted as fuel for other dreams?** These are efforts and ideas that are potent, but didn't survive this year's wind and weather. Luckily, they'll make for nutrient rich soil in which to bury this year's seeds.

### Gratitude Walk

The goal of the gratitude walk is to observe the things you see around you as you walk. Take it all in. Be aware of nature, the colors of the trees, the sounds the birds make, and the smell of the plants. Notice how your feet feel when you step onto the ground.

The effects are more potent when you can enjoy a gratitude walk with your partner or a friend. In this way, you can show them an appreciation for being able to spend the time walking together.

### Gratitude Collage

This is similar to the gratitude journal, except you are going to take pictures of all the things you are grateful for. This gives you the opportunity to visualize your gratitude.

Try taking a picture of one thing you are grateful for every day for a week. Notice how you feel. Take a look back at the pictures every week. You don't have to find grandiose things to be grateful for. A simple picture of a flower will do.

The more you do this the easier it will be for you to spot out the things you are grateful for. You will no longer take these simple things for granted.

Perhaps you will document multiple pictures in a day. After a given time period put all your pictures together in a collage and simply be grateful for all that you have.

~

Now is the time for drying, canning, and storing the past season's bounty. It's also time to put our gardens to bed for the coming winter. Some of my favorite harvest-time tasks are seed collection and storing them away in labeled envelopes for next year's garden. I also love the hours of preparing peaches, pears, and apple slices for the dehydrator. I turn on some music, roll up my sleeves, and allow myself the time and space to enjoy the meditative groove that overtakes me. It's usually during these long-form harvest tasks that my mind and body become creatively unlocked. This is when I am flooded with ideas and impulses for my next creative project.

So often, we expect the muse to arrive only when we have a wide swath of unencumbered time. Or we're told that inspiration strikes only when the artist is properly primed in their solitary studio. But this is not the case. There are as many ways to become creatively unlocked as there are people on this earth. Each of us has our own triggers for creative inspiration and awakening.

**Make a list of all the things that help you feel creatively unlocked— the sources you reach for, the tools you need, the objects that inspire you, the workspace and routines that feel generative.**

**Then, write about what this list reveals about you and your creative process.**

~

It's also important to take creative rest at this time of year. If you've been go-go-going, as I have been, then perhaps we need a moment to step away from harvest chores and pending projects.

Gold is the color of summer's end in Eastern Oregon. The caramel and sepia tones alert me to a kind of botanical exhaustion sweeping the fields. In some places, the harvest party is still going strong, but the sun is slipping away earlier and earlier these days. The waning vegetation offers it's last party tricks: flowers, fruits, and seeds. This time of year makes me think about the parts of my creative life that need rest, quiet, and slumber. Mother nature is sending signals from every direction. It might be time to imitate the action of the sun or follow the lead of the ebbing landscape. Nothing blooms all year.

**Do you feel the ebb of the season making its way into your own energy levels?**

**Which parts of your life are ready for a little rest?**

**What does creative rest look like for you?**

ONE-WORD PROMPTS FOR MABON

Seeds • Surrender • Husk • Oak • Gratitude
Skin • Apple • Enough • Sovereignty • Pod
Offering • Rematriate • Wise • Protect • Limit
Generation • Sunflower • Wane • Indigenous • Inception
Release • Kindling • Cornfield • Reserve • Sunset
Survive • Cornucopia • Quietude • Feast • Transition

THE NEXT SIX WEEKS

Whether you are new to a gratitude practice or have years of experience, take some notes over the next six weeks considering these questions: How does gratitude change how you feel about what you already have? How does gratitude affect your relationships with people, plants, animals, and other fellow travelers on the Creative Alchemy path? What doors does gratitude open? What pain does gratitude ease? What possibilities does gratitude possess? What solutions does gratitude illuminate?

## CROSS THE THRESHOLD

I'm back in Cassie's garden today. Successive nights of frost have laid waste to summer's left-overs. I remove dark ropes of squash vines from the hog fence and till the wide umbrella-like leaves back into the soil. Cassie has already collected the last hurrah of beans and seeds for next year's garden. They're all labeled and filed away in her seed bank, a plastic bucket stuffed full of zip lock baggies and folded paper envelopes.

As I take in the landscape beyond the garden, I see signs that everything is nearing the end of its annual cycle. Trees and flowers, once teeming with life, have gone silent. They now rest in the knowledge that they've set their seeds and completed their work. The only sound is a cawing crow, sitting on the roof of the water pump near the creek. It watches as I put the garden to bed.

Tonight Cassie and Zizi will host a bonfire. They've invited a circle of friends to mark the coming dark by burning last season's debris. But even this ritual marking of time has a practical use. Wood ash contains significant amounts of potassium and calcium and also smaller amounts of phosphorous, magnesium, and micro-nutrients like zinc and copper. Once the fire has cooled, we'll fold the ashes into the soil. A final act of gratitude for this season's abundance.

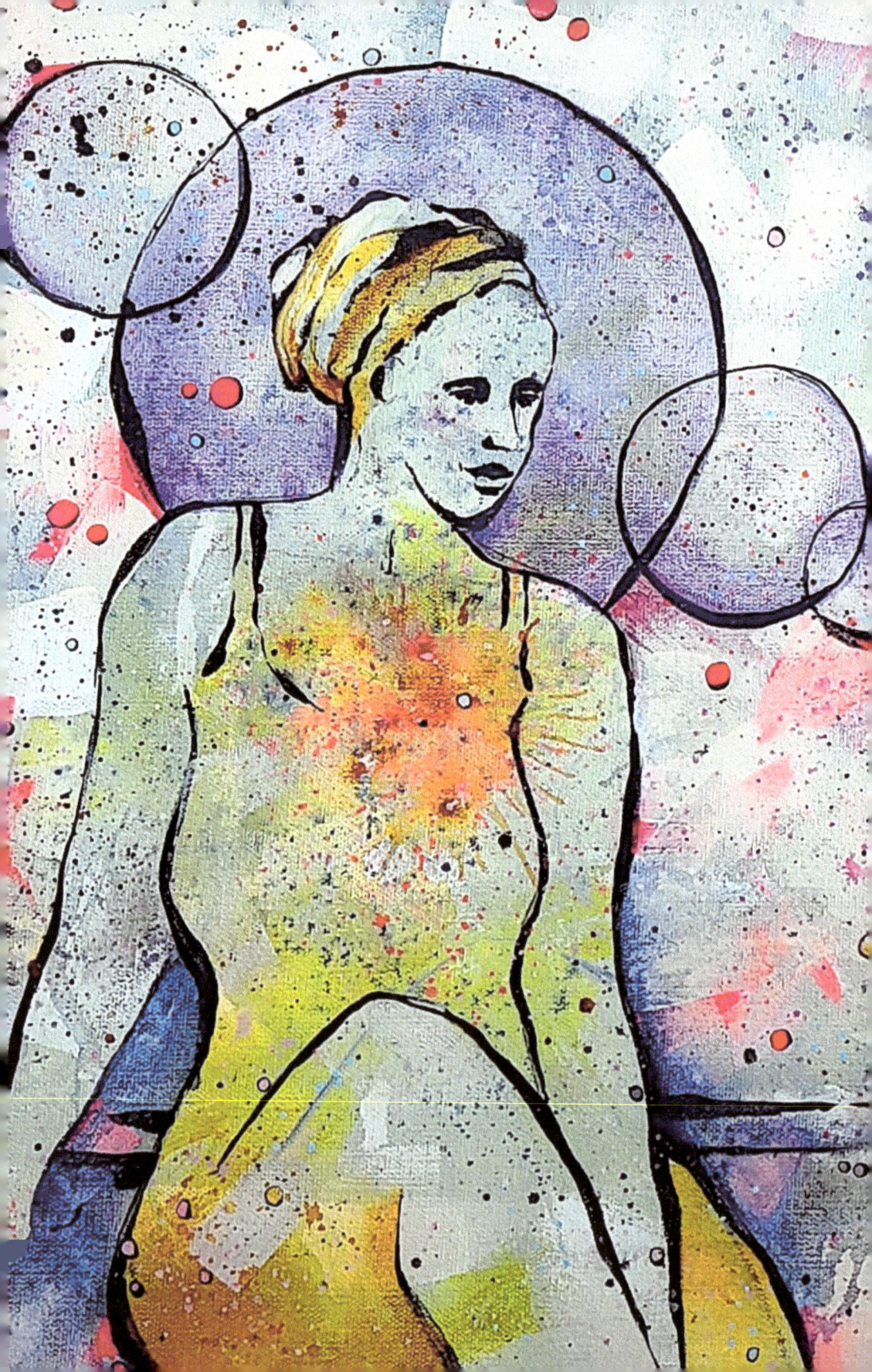

8

---

# WE ARE SHADOWS: SAMHAIN

## GRIEF PRACTICE

**The Call:** Grief is an invitation to become more fully human.

**The Question:** What within me is longing to transform?

**The Time:** October 31 - November 1

**The Origin:** Samhain (pronounced SAH-win) is an ancient Gaelic festival marking the end of harvest and the beginning of the Celtic new year. It also marks the halfway point between the autumn equinox and the winter solstice.

**The Imagery:** Candle, Moon, Owl, Skull, Chalice or Bowl

**The Themes:** Darkness, Spirit Life, Transition

IT'S TIME TO PEER INTO THE SHADOWS AND WELCOME THE COMING DARK. Samhain invites us to celebrate mystery, honor our quiet creative time, and make some space for our darker emotional cosmology. This moment may challenge you to appreciate the fallow times that must follow the abundant ones. The void itself is a creative fertile space.

Grief work can bring up all sorts of painful memories and present realities. Please know that whatever your history, whatever your trespasses, whatever wounds you've spent your life nursing — you are worthy of love and healing. In this chapter, you are invited to breathe into the center of your secret grief and trust your creativity to work its alchemical magic. Let grief share its gifts and move through you. This is how we step out of the shadow and into the light. Look up. Feel the late autumn sun on your face. Healing is possible.

Sometimes we find ourselves battling our inner critic (I call mine the shitty committee) or fighting against old stories we've heard from others or absorbed from our environment. One of the most tangible, effective, and joyful ways I know to de-fang the harmful inner narratives that hold my mind hostage is a creative practice rooted in reverence for Earth's seasonal cycles. I journal. I paint. I sew. I arrange natural objects on my window sill. I make music. My creative practice calms me, heals me, and welcomes me home. Every time.

You are invited to allow the tender parts of your body to adapt to new information. Receive the gift of silence and solitude. You don't have to know it all or do it all. Especially all at once. Welcome the drip-drop of knowing as it pools up inside of you. Inner work must happen first before it is made manifest with outward action. There is no urgency. Only the potent and powerful moment before you.

CALLING YOU HOME – A SEASONAL HOMILY FOR SAMHAIN

It's October now and the wind is biting back. Sundown comes earlier and earlier as I watch the temperature gauge on my back porch take its nightly dive. The slow fading sunsets of late summer have surrendered to autumn nights that come on fast and have a growing animated energy that feels alive and purposeful. My sense of hearing is turned up at this time of year, as the expanding darkness invites all things nocturnal out into the open. I cannot see, but I can hear.

Every autumn, a great horned owl takes up residence atop the Douglas fir outside my studio door. Each morning, I go outside to find little mummified mice skeletons swaddled along with other indigestible bits of bone, claws, fur, and feathers. Each night around 7pm I hear his low throaty hoot. But sometimes, in the witching hours, he screams.

When I first moved to Eastern Oregon, his screech startled me, and arrested my body where it stood. It mimicked what I imagine the cry of a banshee (*bean sídhe*) might sound like. But now, as I have grown more accustomed to his presence, the owl's lament is a kind of comfort.

As a child, I remember my grandmother reading to me from a thick volume with a yellow jacket cover called *An Encyclopedia of Fairies : Hobgoblins, Brownies, Bogies, and Other Supernatural Creatures*. The section devoted to the *bean sídhe* was my favorite. Depicted as a weeping wraith, jaw unhinged, raw with emotion, she filled me with both terror and deep curiosity. Also empathy. To hear the cry and keen of the *bean sídhe* was an omen of death.

In Celtic lore, Samhain offers the *bean sídhe* and faerie folk of all ilks an opportunity to come out for a night to wander the countryside. It's also the one night of the year that the dead revisit their mortal homes. Families lay out offerings of food and set great bonfires to light the way from house to house.

This year for Samhain, I'm setting a place of honor at our table for my brother Joel. His accidental death at the cold hands of oxycontin laid me bare. And in the wake of his death came a myriad of feelings: confusion, pain, rage. At the time, I had great need of some kind of container to hold my grief. I needed a place to mourn. I needed a way to honor this big feeling that rocked my body and left me completely undone by its magnitude and power. I needed a way to sing my brother's soul home... to sing my own soul home.

Some take their pain to church. And while that works well for many, it isn't quite right for me. I was raised Methodist and the funerals of my youth were quiet, reverent, stoic, and over in about an hour. I wanted a place to take my *real* grief – my 'screaming in the car on the highway' grief, my 'sobbing in the public bathroom at a Walmart' grief, my 'horrific accusations to the dead soul of my brother shouted into the night sky' grief. I felt like the *bean sídhe* from grandma's Encyclopedia, keening and wailing my song for the dead under cover of night, scaring the neighbors and starting rumors about my mental stability.

Keening is a very old Irish rite – a powerful, poetic, public, and ritualized lamentation for the dead. The word keen comes from the Gaelic *caoineadh*, to weep or cry. The *bean chaointe* was a woman who specialized in embodied transformational, ritualized grieving.

When Christianity came to the Celtic lands, keening was banned. Who needs the *bean chaointe* when you have a priest to now escort the souls of the dead over the threshold?

The thing I love about keening is that it contains not only the grief of the loss of a single loved one, but also holds the passionate rage - female rage in particular - of the society at large. It is said that keeners inhabit the emotional and spiritual borderlands.

They traveled not on the highways, but rather through the wilderness, barefoot, and often in a state of disheveled undress. She was *other*. Separate. Her ability to be in and of the earth, so close to nature, gave her direct access to the liminal space between the world of the living and the dead. She cut herself off from the community at large because of her unstable and surprising behavior, and yet gained license to speak truth with passion, rage, and clarity. She was seen as holy.

The art of keening, once an integral part of the Irish grieving process, began to vanish in the early 1800's. Perhaps it was because of the modernization of Irish life during the industrial revolution. Perhaps it was because keening was in direct conflict with the Christian church.

I think of my great-great grandmothers living in Ireland at the time – Glennah Gertrude Dulin, Lillie Celeste Bailey, and Mary Wilks Minshull. They must have heard the keeners as children. Perhaps they even participated themselves. I often wonder if they invited the *bean chaointe* to come keen for their stillbirths and dead sons of war. I imagine them arriving, wild and barefooted from the forest. Bridges to the otherworld. Perhaps they'd wail and sing outside the homes of my ancestors, giving their grief voice.

I imagine the neighbors listening in, laying their hands on their hearts in a gesture of recognition. Perhaps they understood that some grief is too big for one body to carry alone. Perhaps they knew that some kinds of grief require the whole community. What a gift the keeners gave. They held the enormous pain of my family and sang it aloud. The keeners were there to lead us through the labyrinth of loss and sing us home.

For the Celtic people, death was a moment of outward release. There was no disenfranchised grieving - just grieving. Loss was loss and those who mourned were considered holy. Keening was a palpable way to recognize the sacred mystery of death and honor the great unknown.

Keening as a community practice is no more, but I long for a replacement. Until then, I make art. It seems simple and stupid in the face of something as complex and unwieldy as grief. But I think it helps. I paint. I sing. I knit. I write. Not for the product I make at the end, but for the process. For the doing of it.

When I close my eyes and think about the countless stone circles that dot the Irish and Scottish landscape, all aligned to the sun and stars, I see that my people were well aware of the necessity to preserve a universal perspective of death and lamentation.

This Samhain, we continue to celebrate the darker half of the year and grieve the dying light. And we find ourselves once again at the intersection of the material and the spiritual. So pull out the photo of a loved one dead and gone. Set an extra plate at the table for an ancestor. Light a candle to help your body remember. You do not have to carry this alone. Samhain invites us to hold the enormity and bear witness together.

And while this creative threshold may feel disorienting, it is the perfect time for transformational magic and inviting your inner wisdom to take center stage. Ask yourself: "What within me is longing to transform?"

Sylvia Townsend Warner tells us "to shed oneself downward like a tree, to be almost wholly earth before one dies." Samhain asks that we place the things we value at the center of our lives. Then make their nourishment, attention, and stewardship the business of our everyday living. Everything else is dust.

Strip yourself.
Shed downward.
Get low.
Remember you are Earth.

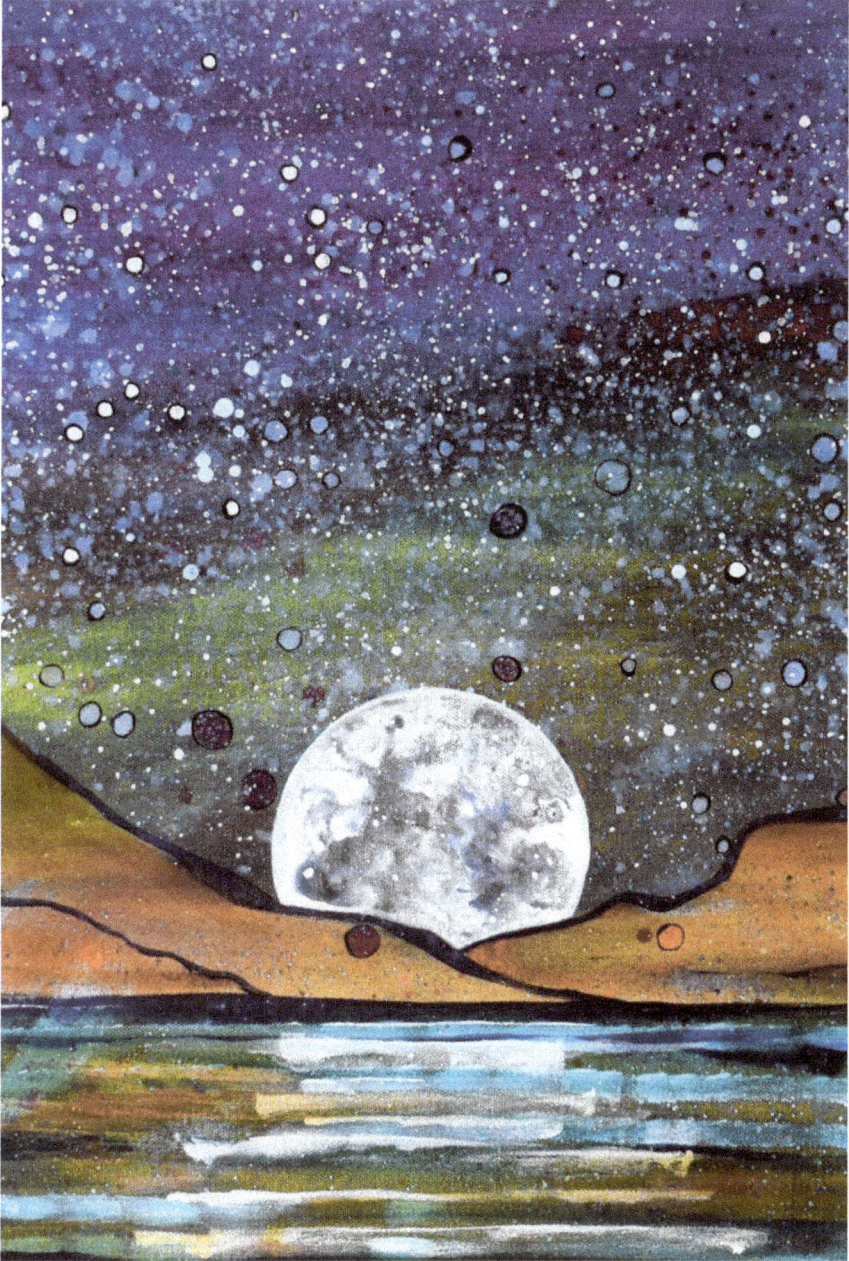

TEND THE ALTAR

The full moon hangs heavy in the sky tonight. And as she gazes down on Earth's northern hemisphere, she'll surely see the tell-tale rust-gold of autumn sweeping the land. Here in Eastern Oregon, the leaves are in their final moments. Soon, the trees will be bare.

It doesn't matter how many times I witness the phenomenon of falling leaves, I'm still struck by the sheer magic of it all. *Abscission* is a biological function that describes the shedding of various parts of an organism, such as a plant dropping a leaf, fruit, flower, or seed. In zoology, *abscission* is the intentional shedding of a body part, such as the shedding of a claw, husk, or antler. But tonight, backlit by the full moon, I watch the leaves release their hold on life and one-by-one, fall to the ground.

During this moment on the Wheel of the Year, there is a kind of spiritual understanding to be gained from engaging the sacred darkness that Earth has on offer. It can be found in the falling leaves, the waning light, the bitter winds, and the trees drawing back their life force and burying it deep in their roots for the winter to come. It is a liminal time and there are thresholds everywhere for those who wish to cross them.

I live at the edge of a great wood called the Eagle Cap Wilderness. Here, the valley floor is flanked by thick stands of Ponderosa and Aspen. I've stood in the fields and watched deer and elk disappear and appear out of the forest wall. Biologists call spaces like this "ecotones" — biological edges, where two different systems meet and are places of great dynamism and tension. But they are also the places for enhanced creativity and diversity. These liminal places create a kind of third system that is often richer and more vital than the other two alone. This is also true for systems of thought. Bringing together two ideas to create a third more potent iteration of the original two, for instance spirituality and ecology or creativity and seasonality.

The season of Samhain (pronounced SAH-win) is upon us — an ancient Gaelic festival marking the end of harvest and the beginning of the Celtic new year. Samhain begins on the evening of October 31st, and ends on the evening of November 1st. At this time, it is believed that the veil between this earthly world and the otherworld is at its thinnest. Samhain is a fire festival that honors the ancestors. It's also the perfect time for transformational magic, for standing at the edge of your experience and inviting your inner wisdom to take center stage.

The Celts have a visceral understanding of what they call the otherworld. This is not the underworld, where Persephone is on the throne ruling over the land of the dead. Rather, the otherworld is this realm of the Sidhe, as they are known in Ireland, or Sìth, as they are known in Scotland. Both Sidhe and Sìth are pronounced as *shee*. The otherworld has infiltrated the popular imagination through the lens of fairy tales from the Brothers Grimm all the way to Steven Sondheim's *Into The Woods*. In the modern era, we see it as mythology. But for Celtic people, the otherworld is a reality — a world that exists alongside our own. Human beings tend to focus on a physical experience of the world while the Sidhe are rooted in the spiritual or the conscious. The place where these two worlds intersect is its own kind of ecotone — its own kind of spiritual edge. And it is during Samhain, the historical precursor for Halloween, that the space between is most porous.

So why cross the veil and engage the otherworld? For me, my Celtic ancestors built their entire lives, their stories, relationships, and work around a truth — not a mythology — that the otherworld exists alongside ours. And the woods, the wildernesses, the forests, these are threshold places that hold wisdom, mystery, and are the gateway to the otherworld.

And it's not just an external wilderness that acts as a threshold for consciousness. There is also an internal wilderness— a wild landscape inside of each human soul. It's an internal landscape where we are still wholly wild, connected to the earth, animistic, and free. But as we've moved into the modern era and been domesticated, we've forgotten that inner wilderness. The Celts call it a kind of 'Soul-Forgetting'. And

Samhain season offers an opportunity to peer through the veil and remember. Collective remembering.

Autumn is always a time of grieving for me. Or perhaps it might be better described as "griefs remembered." This time of year marks the ecological descent into winter and it comes on the heels of many difficult private anniversaries of the heart. But I also love this time of year because it offers a transitional moment of decay as an opportunity to face some of my darker emotions.

This particular season, I have been processing a lot of anger and hurt. I don't like being angry. And I'm not very good at it. So, as a protective measure, I pretend that it's not happening. I've been carefully taught to do this (as so many women are) — taught first that I'm wrong in my perceptions and therefore wrong to feel as I do. It takes time to release this kind of pretending.

The poet Rumi tells us, "Be like a tree and let the dead leaves drop." As I age and step into the power of my mid-40s, I feel called to name harm and burn down the structures that maintained my silence and my obedience. This is happening for me in both perceptible and invisible ways. My creative work now is to transmute that anger into something generative and healing. To alchemize it. This is at the heart of the Creative Alchemy Cycle: to recognize the grief we carry, to give it voice and power through the creative act, to invite it to move through us. Grief as creative partner.

Today, as the leaves drop and cover the land and model their ancient process of *abscission* to all who bear witness, I am inspired to release false protection. If we can't show up in our fullness, then we can't do the soul-work we're meant to do.

Trees that hang on to dead leaves create more surface area for winter snow to accumulate. Snow is heavy and the tree ends up losing limbs instead of just leaves. So this season, I'm focusing on letting the dead leaves drop.

The work I've identified for myself as an artist is to create a context that supports and honors grieving. I believe that the gift of grief is that it is deeply humanizing. Terry Tempest Williams writes, "There is deep beauty in not averting our gaze." Bearing witness to grief, holding its gaze, and allowing it to reveal its gifts, is the key to alchemizing the pain into connection and yes, even joy. This doesn't mean that the grief goes away. Rather, it has the potential to be your co-creator in getting free.

This season, we'll use our creative gifts to walk to the edge of the field and step into the wood before us. With storytelling, meaning-making, art, and ritual, we'll explore the emotional ecotone that marries light and shadow. We'll tenderly hold our grief, roll it around in our hands, and examine it through the lens of curiosity, creativity, and gratitude. Perhaps we might even befriend our grief and allow it to fuel a new form of healing. What might that look or feel like?

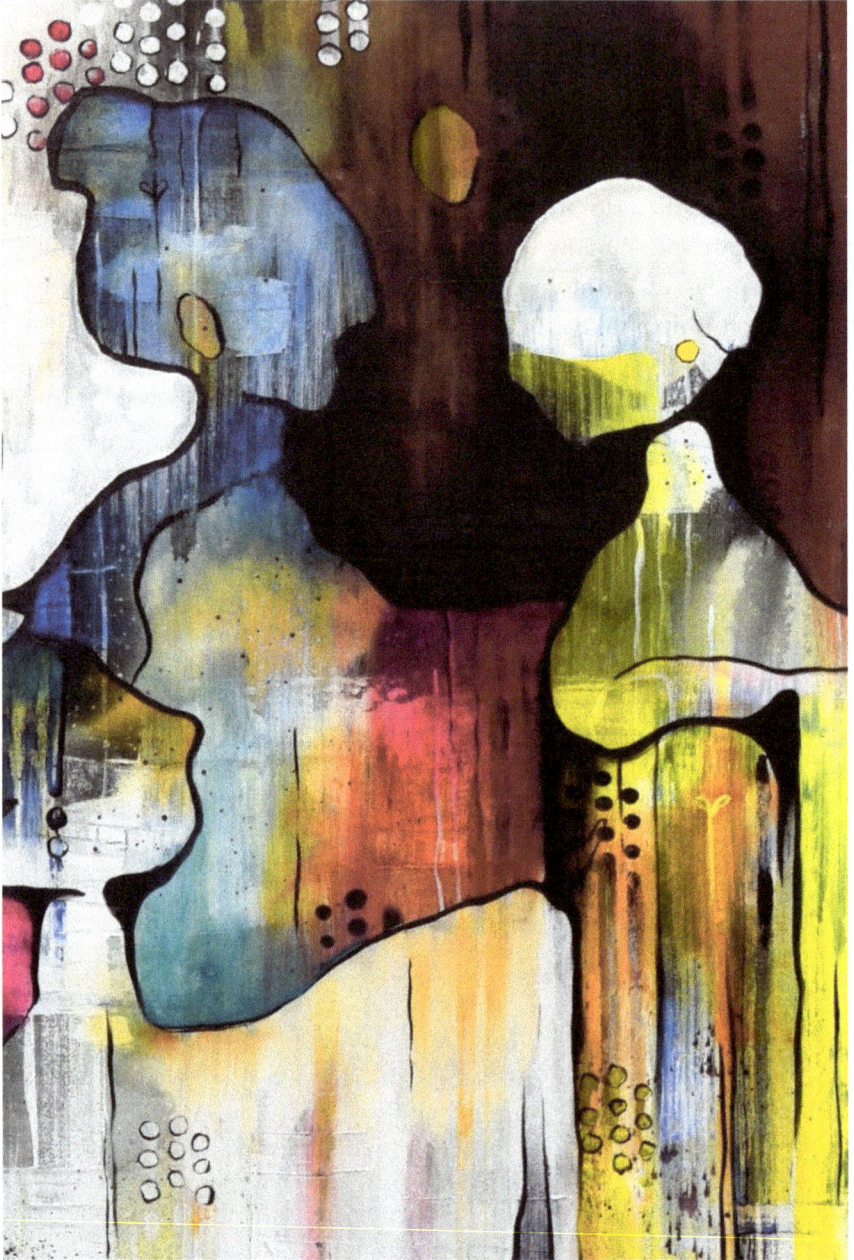

GRIEF PRACTICE

Ritual is a potent form of creativity that can help access these liminal spaces and shed light inside the shadows. But before we dive in, I want to share some thoughts on tenderness as we enter into this work. Grief requires intentional tenderness. As we journal, story tell and weave ritual into our creative process, you are invited to hold, with both hands, your tender heart and your tender body. Receive yourself with tenderness. And receive others with tenderness. Let it inform all of your interactions and actions. Tenderness is never a lie. Never a false promise. It is always purely itself. An antidote for distraction, dissociation, and broken-heartedness. Allow yourself to be enveloped by the truth it offers. And if at any time, you feel that a story, or an ache, or a sorrow is too hot to touch, then please take care of yourself and let it be. If however, you feel the urge to hold it and work with it, do it tenderly.

～

This time of year invites us to celebrate mystery, creative incubation, and the shadow self. And we don't have to look far to see naturally occurring signs of Samhain's seasonal magic. Every once in a while, the Earth experiences a Penumbral Lunar Eclipse. Full lunar eclipses can only occur during a full moon, but a penumbral lunar eclipse is different from a total lunar eclipse. A penumbral eclipse occurs when the moon moves into Earth's penumbra, or outer shadow. This causes the moon to look darker than normal.

What a great word, right? "Penumbra" took on new meaning for me when I watched *What the Constitution Means to Me*, a play written and performed by Heidi Schreck. "Here I am, standing in the light," Schreck says from the front of the stage, "and there you are, sitting in the darkness. This space between us, this space right here of partial illumination, this shadowy space right here: This is the penumbra."

Schreck continues, "Penumbra" is how Supreme Court Justice William O. Douglas described the Ninth Amendment — the murkiest and least understood part of the constitution, even for Supreme Court Justices. (Justice Scalia once said he didn't even remember studying it in school.) But it's the amendment that leaves room to find new rights, that states that "just because a certain right is not listed in the constitution, it doesn't mean you don't have that right."

I love the idea of a penumbra because it means there exists, in the shadows of our certainties, a space of not only possibility, but also unlearned truths, rights, and collective knowledge — already present and ready for our future self to discover. This idea is most potent during the shadow season of Samhain.

**What truths and bits of wisdom exist in the shadows of our experiences?**

**And how do we access our own penumbra and make the invisible visible?**

## INCUBATION

Grief is often processed in a solitary way. Sure, there are times when we need to hold it in a community context, as the keeners once did. But often, we find ourselves holding it in solitude. Solitude is a gift you give to yourself. It's different from loneliness or isolation. Solitude is a generative, creative state of being, where you are able to listen to the inner stirrings of your deepest desires. Carve some time out of your schedule this week or next and spend a few hours alone. Let's give ourselves some air. Pack your favorite snacks, wear comfortable clothes, and attend to the needs of your inner life. And if you don't have an hour, perhaps consider twenty minutes or even ten. It's okay to start with small intervals of time. Anne Morrow Lindberg reminds us that "certain springs are tapped only when we are alone." And many of the writing and ritual prompts on offer this season are best done in a state of solitude, however momentary it might be.

ACTION

One of the most potent ways I infuse my work with magic and energy at this time of year is to make Full Moon and Lunar Eclipse Water. It is both a form of ritual nourishment and also a tangible way to welcome edge-dweller energy. For me, making moon water helps me capture the creative energy of shadow, of darkness, and of grief and transform it into a tool for healing.

When you have a moment, check your calendar for the next full moon. And also take note if there happens to be a lunar eclipse. Full moons and eclipses are a wonderful opportunity to capture the essence of their energy and wisdom. We'll be making Full Moon Water (or Lunar Eclipse Water if we happen to find one on the calendar) so that we can put it to future use as a way of opening ourselves to yet-known truths. The purpose of this ritual is to bottle up all that good energy and use it for months after the event has passed.

**What you'll need:**

A clear container with a lid. I typically use a mason jar.

Water. I use tap water, but feel free to use filtered water if you prefer.

**What you'll do:**

Fill up your clear container with water and close it tight.

Set your mason jar out under the full moon and make sure it stays out for the penumbral lunar eclipse. (Tip: If you're using a Mason jar, flip it upside down so the lid is on the bottom. Then the Moon energy can shine in through the glass.)

While your water is collecting energy, set your intention.

Put your water away once the lunar eclipse is complete.

**How you can use your moon water (the possibilities are endless):**

Apply it to your Third Eye Chakra to enhance meditation or psychic awareness.

I like to use my moon water for watercolor painting.

Put some in your drinking water when you need power, luck, or help for the day. I also like to drink a bit before I sit down to write in my journal. This can be especially potent when I'm writing about grief, as I often do during Samhain.

Add to ice cube trays and use them in your drinks. You can also add some herbs or flowers of choice based on your intentions.

Use it to bake when you're making something extra special.

Wash your face with it for luminosity and revival. This is also a way to honor your skin as you age.

Add to a spray bottle for cleaning your home. Mix white vinegar and moon water in a 50/50 mix. Add orange, lemon peels, rosemary, lavender, or whatever you choose. Great for cleansing, protection, and purifying your home.

Use it to water your plants when they're looking down.

Use it in a humidifier and infuse your air with its energy.

Keep a small bottle, vial, or container of it with you during your daily routine. This will allow you to keep the Moon water energy with you all day. It can also act as a kind of happiness/positivity jar.

Add it to other plant essences to magnify their effect.

Put it in your coffee maker for an extra boost of energy.

Mix it with warm water and Epsom salt for a foot bath to remember.

Add some peppermint essential oil to your Moon Water and wipe down doors and windows. Not only does it keep out negative energy but bugs as well!

Add some to your animal's water bowl when they're feeling sick or lonely.

～

The following creative prompts are geared towards developing our relationship with grief and healing. They are not triggering by nature, but they may be emotionally difficult for those of us who've experienced serious trauma. This is not therapy, but rather a means of creative excavation. My intention is always a deeper understanding of our own lived human experiences as a pathway towards collective liberation.

In his book, *Courting the Wild Twin*, Martin Shaw introduces readers to the idea that our ancestors, or as he calls them the old ones, are communicating to us through time and space and age and earth. During Samhain season, the veil between the worlds is thin and we have an opportunity to connect to these cues, messages, and missives from the otherworld. They come in the form of awakenings, bits of wisdom read, heard, or remembered. And sometimes they come in more mysterious ways: in the form of dreams, inspiration, mental states of flow or chaos.

Shaw writes, "The earth has scattered many clues around you so you pick up their scent. But who are the old ones? They are your invested dead… they are the whole bright universe talking to you."

**Who are the "old ones" in your life?**

**How do they communicate with you?**

**How do they help you to honor and hold your grief?**

In my seasonal homilies, I write in a style that is considered creative nonfiction. As a memoirist, there is always a moment when I come to a dead end in my writing. It usually happens when I want to explore something that I don't have any "real" information about. In the case of my Homily for Samhain, which I shared at the beginning of this chapter, I wanted to explore how my great-great grandmothers may have handled their grief given the likelihood that they had knowledge of and access to Irish "keening" rituals.

In Lisa Knopp's essay "Perhapsing: The Use of Speculation in Creative Nonfiction", she describes how a writer can use phrases like "perhaps", "maybe", "might have", and "what if" to mine the unknown parts of our stories. Knopp writes, "'Perhapsing' can be particularly useful when writing about childhood memories, which are often incomplete because of a child's limited understanding at the time of the event, and the loss of the details and clarity due to the passage of time."

**Make a list of memories you have about your mother or grandmother (or any other relative of importance to you) in which their motivation was not clear to you. If you didn't know your mother or grandmother, begin by writing the facts and details that you do know.**

**Pick one of these moments and free-write for 15 minutes. Let yourself speculate using "perhaps" or "maybe" or "I wonder".**

**After you are finished, read what you've written. Did you open a new window of perspective?**

**For those of you who'd like to dive deeper into this exercise, take your free-write and turn it into a first person monologue from the point of view of your mother or grandmother as I did with my homily. Let your mother or grandmother tell the story of your memory from her own perspective.**

**You can repeat this process with as many relations as you like.**

INTEGRATION

As I move more fully into my 40s, I find myself shedding the "shoulds" of my 20s and 30s. A small example: I stopped wearing make-up and dying my hair two years ago. While it may seem like an insignificant way of letting go, it has been truly liberating to disengage from the beauty machine. Now I appear to be as I am: a woman in my 40s, unapologetic, claiming space and owning my lived experience.

Perhaps you've had a similar experience? Perhaps as you move forward with life and let go of old ways of being, you may find an under layer of grief that needs to be released as well. Embrace this era of aging and shedding with curiosity, conviction, and courage. Lift off. Ruin your reputation. Where you once sought acceptance and admission, seek mischief and magic. Live in the penumbra of your experience and live it on your own terms: natural, un-dyed, raw, present, and in our power. Remember who you've always been: your own muse.

Here are some questions for your journal:

**What are you shedding as you age?**

**What old narratives no longer serve you?**

**Have you experienced grief as you change and release old parts of yourself? How does it manifest?**

**As you age, what kind of good mischief are you willing to get into in service of your freedom and the freedom of those around you?**

## ONE-WORD PROMPTS FOR SAMHAIN

Shadow • Soul • Decay • Listen • Ghost
Bones • Pomegranate • Descend • Ache • Ashes
Weave • Ancestor • Nocturnal • Dreamscape • Ebb
Compost • Sage • Remember • Medicine • Silence
Bare • Age • Release • Banshee • Penumbra
Lunar • Secret • Grave • Liminal • Mystery

## THE NEXT SIX WEEKS

The writer Ellen Bass is a master at using poetry to examine grief. In her poem called *The Thing Is,* she writes about a moment we all know well when "everything you've held dear crumbles like burnt paper in your hands." Navigating grief and loss is one of the key markers of the human experience. And we are generally unpracticed at holding grief – for ourselves and for others. The darkening days between Samhain and Yule are often full of end of year activities and holidays of all sorts. But they are also a time of memory and absence. In this quiet season of shadow and decay, allow the prompts and rituals in this chapter to be a catalyst for continued self-inquiry, processing and healing.

## CROSS THE THRESHOLD

Samhain invites you to set a place at the table for your grief. Give it welcome. This season, you and thousands of mourners like you, will make offerings of bread and wine and decorate their mantles with flowers, fruit, full moon water, and photos of loved ones who've passed on.

As we settle our souls and comfort our grief-stricken, inner selves, we ask for and receive grace. Grace can come in many forms: breath, song, space, solitude. It's not easy to become whole. So, we stand together embracing the wisdom that Samhain offers. Cross the threshold of your experience. Dance in the penumbra. Explore your learning edge. Stand once more at the precipice of your own healing. Become yourself again.

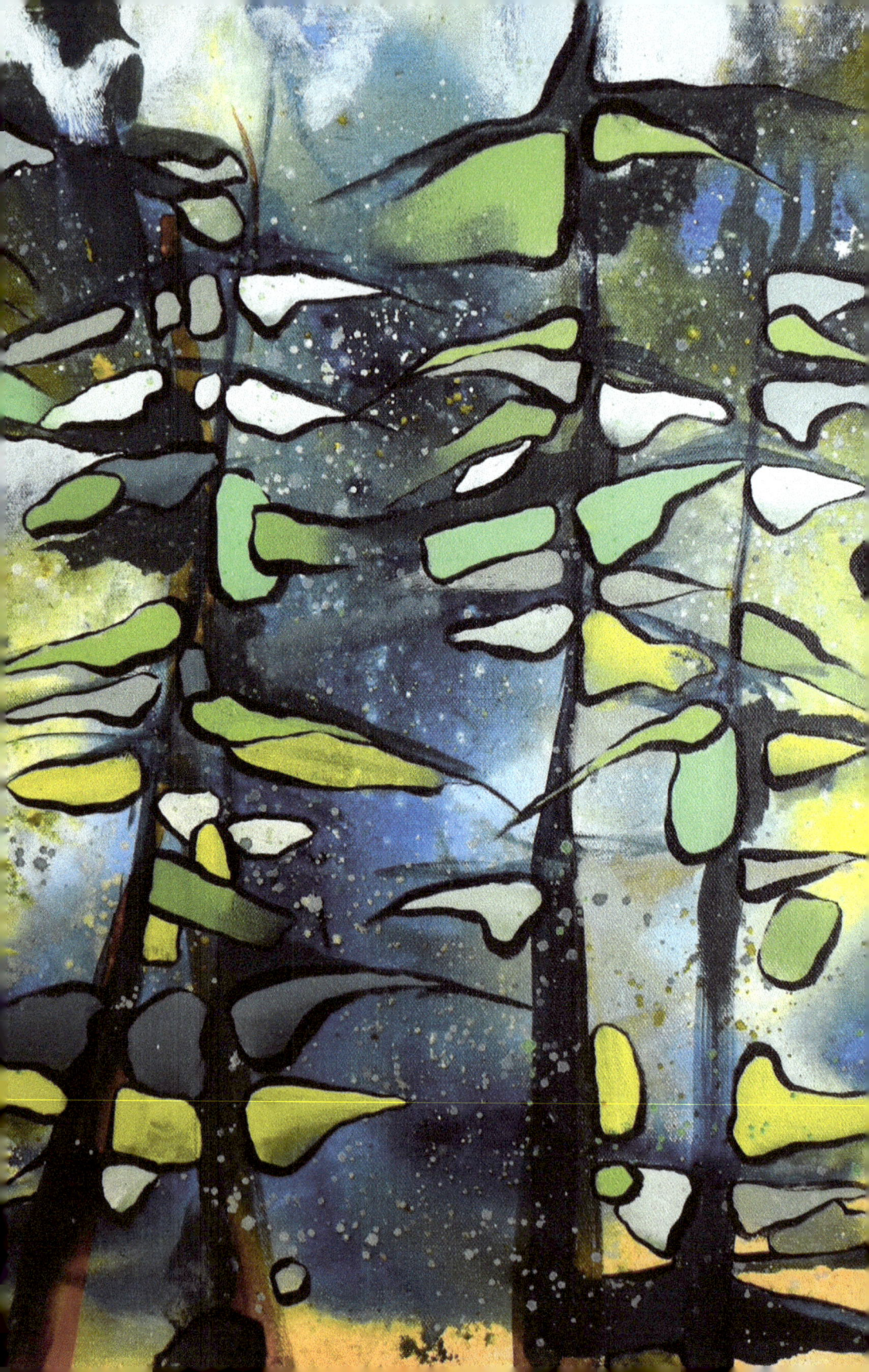

# 9

# WE ARE LIGHT: YULE

## JOY PRACTICE

**The Call:** Let your light shine.

**The Question:** What might occur if I truly shared my creative gifts with the world?

**The Time:** December 19-21

**The Origin:** Yule (pronounced YOOL) marks the longest night of the year.

**The Imagery:** Pinecone, Candle, Conifer, Sun, Star, Wreath

**The Themes:** Illumination, Reflection, Transformation, Homecoming

THE WINTER SOLSTICE, KNOWN IN CELTIC CULTURE AS YULE, MARKS THE return of the sun. It's called the 'season of light' for a reason. For those of us in the northern hemisphere, Yule occurs sometime between December 20 and 22. This ancient holiday is observed by most religious traditions and honors the solar return, highlighting themes of rebirth, active hope, intention-setting, illumination and enlightenment. So soak it in, friends. The season of Yule is upon us! Joy. Joy. Joy.

As light returns, we give thanks for the darkness. We give thanks for the creeks as they ice over, thanks for the howling Coyotes prowling the foothills, thanks for the feisty birds elbowing each other at the edge of the birdfeeder, thanks for the hearth that heats the bones of our homes, and thanks for all the silence that surrounds us. I wonder if these winter gifts were what the composer Issac Watts was referring to when he wrote "repeat the sounding joy." Let's all share the gifts of our grateful hearts as we dive into our creative work this season. Then might we truly deliver joy to the world.

CALLING YOU HOME — A SEASONAL HOMILY FOR YULE

Everyone said it was a terrible time of year for a cross-country move. A well-meaning neighbor wrinkled her nose when we shared our plan. "Mid-December? You do realize it snows here, right?" As far as she knew, we were Texas rookies. Unpracticed. What did we know of heavy snow-fall, frozen pipes, and icy road conditions?

We arrived at Pine Cottage just days ahead of the Winter Solstice. Our U-Haul caravan had taken us from Texas to New Mexico, through Colorado, up to Wyoming, across Idaho, and into Eastern Oregon. And aside from a little black ice along Highway 80, it was smooth sailing.

We pulled up to the house and tumbled out of the van. The air smelled of fir needles and pine resin. Heaven. Katie, my oldest child, went bounding like a filly through the front gate and kicked a pine cone from the walkway. She twirled around, eyes toward the bright white sky. "Look at these trees! They're huge!" For a kid born and bred in Texas, these trees might as well have been the Great Pyramids of Giza.

Our home was built in 1925. It is situated on a large corner lot encircled by Douglas fir trees with twin Norway conifers that anchor the street corner. They're all squished together at the edge of our property, suffocated by the road, our house, and each other, popping out thousands of pine cones every year in hopes of reproducing on the inhospitable gravel road below.

Most folks around here grow produce or raise livestock. When asked if we farm, Katie jokes that we raise pine cones. I wish there was a market for them. Seriously, we'd make a killing.

Conifers are some of the oldest forms of plant life on earth. In fact they go back 300 million years. That means they've existed nearly three times longer than all flowering plant species. They've survived countless ages of fire and ice because of their incredible adaptive features -- their bio-plasticity. They are cone-shaped, with flexible branches which help them to cope with heavy snowfall. Their thin waxy needles reduce water loss. And their evergreen nature means that the needles can photosynthesize whenever there is sufficient sunlight. (Please let me return to earth in my next life as a pine tree.)

But to me, the most miraculous part of the tree is the pine cone, an ingenious light-sensitive, sun-worshiping structure perfectly designed to protect and distribute its seeds. The pine cone has long been a symbol of enlightenment and regeneration. And the fact that our new house, the home that would shelter our dreaming, our loving, and our living, was surrounded by pine trees gave me a deep sense of safety and hope.

What's so special about the pine cone that it is a sign of enlightenment and illumination? Have you ever heard of the Pineal gland? It gets its name because it is shaped very much like the pinecone.

You don't mind if I take a little neurology detour here, do you?

So, the "Pine"al gland is a remarkable feature of the human experience. Nestled in the brain between the two hemispheres, it is a source of endless intrigue in the realm of mysticism and science. The Pineal gland is long considered our biological third eye and "the epicenter of enlightenment." Some call it the "dream center" or my favorite, the "mystic seed."

Our Pineal Gland is intimately linked to our body's perception of light and modulates our circadian rhythms. From a purely biological perspective, the pineal gland is integral to the production of melatonin, which is a hormone that facilitates our wake-sleep patterns. In short, it regulates the natural rhythms of sleep according to the presence or lack of light in our environment.

I find it utterly fascinating that the pinecone and Pineal gland share similarities in appearance, but they are also both keenly affected by light. Cones open themselves to the sun's rays, and close during cloudy, darker days. I suppose it has to do with the continuation of the seed-line. Sunny days offer more arid conditions and the tiny seedlings nestled in the scales of the pinecone can become airborne more easily. Damp days are less suitable for spreading seeds. And the Pineal gland is doing the same thing as a function of regulating our body's rhythm.

I never thought neurology would be a passion of mine or that I'd be so continually astonished by the functions of the brain. But then again, I never thought I'd have a child like Charlie.

The first picture of Charlie I ever saw was an MRI. Charlie had been in the NICU for less than 24 hours and was having seizures. Lots of them. My husband and I peered into the muddy scan. The right hemisphere was dark. Nothing. Just a black sea of question marks.

"Brain hemorrhage." The doctor said it as if he was ordering a sandwich. Charlie had suffered a stroke in utero. The doctor dated it at ten days old.

Those first pictures of Charlie's tiny beautiful brain were copied and reproduced and sent ahead to all of his specialists. Like an actor's headshot in a program of a play we had yet to see, these images preceded him and shaped all of his first interactions with the world.

It's amazing, really, that we can see all the little brainy bits and bobs stuffed inside the tiny skull of a newborn. My husband and I were in shock, but riveted as the doctor continued.

"The bleed is in the right parietal lobe. This is the part of the brain that oversees language acquisition, visual processing, stuff like that. He's also lost most of his corpus callosum."

My confused look prompted further explanation, "It's a large C-shaped nerve fiber bundle found beneath the cerebral cortex in the middle of the brain that connects the left and right cerebral hemispheres. It's really the motherboard of the brain, helping the two sides to talk to each other. So it's likely that he'll never talk. And he might be deaf or blind. Or both." And on that sandwich, please hold the tomato, mustard, and onion. Oh and add bacon and avocado. Yes please, both.

After hearing about the extensive damage and learning what it meant to categorize a stroke as "grade four", I asked which parts of the brain were still intact and what that might mean for Charlie's future quality of life.

The doctor forced a smile. "Well, the Cerebellum is untouched. This is the part of the brain that manages coordination and balance. So he may be able to sit up someday. But walking is probably not possible. And also the Pineal Gland is free from the bleed." The doctor perked up. "That's good news", he said looking at his watch.

He didn't go into the details of why it was good news that day. But I knew why. If the Pineal gland was unharmed by the hemorrhage, then Charlie would be able to sleep. And if he could sleep, his cells could regenerate. And if his cells could regenerate, then he could heal.

We humans like to think that we're so different from plants and other naturally occurring earth-bound elements. But we're not. We are dependent on our ecosystems. That's a good thing. We, in fact, are the natural world – not separate from it.

How fitting that our new home is surrounded by pine trees. How perfect that they are constantly dropping cones in our yard. These wise old earth-bound trees are literally throwing symbols of illumination and enlightenment at our family all year long.

And Charlie? Charlie is like these pines. Despite their suffocated root system, poor placement, overlapping branches, they are adapting, resilient, and ever open to the light. If you spend even an hour with Charlie, you'll see that he is indeed a light-bound, light-affected, light-worshiping child. Always drawn to the luminous personality and the warm hug. Always singing the spirit song and the praises of nature.

I remember so clearly, a feeling of active hope, arriving at our new home on that mid-December day. While Katie twirled under the pines, and shouted in praise of their enormity, I helped Charlie step out of the van. I slipped my hands under his armpits to support his weight. He unfurled his legs and stood up. And like all light-susceptible life forms, he lifted his face toward the winter sun, inhaled the pine scent, and said "more."

His first and favorite word: More.
More life. More light. More love.

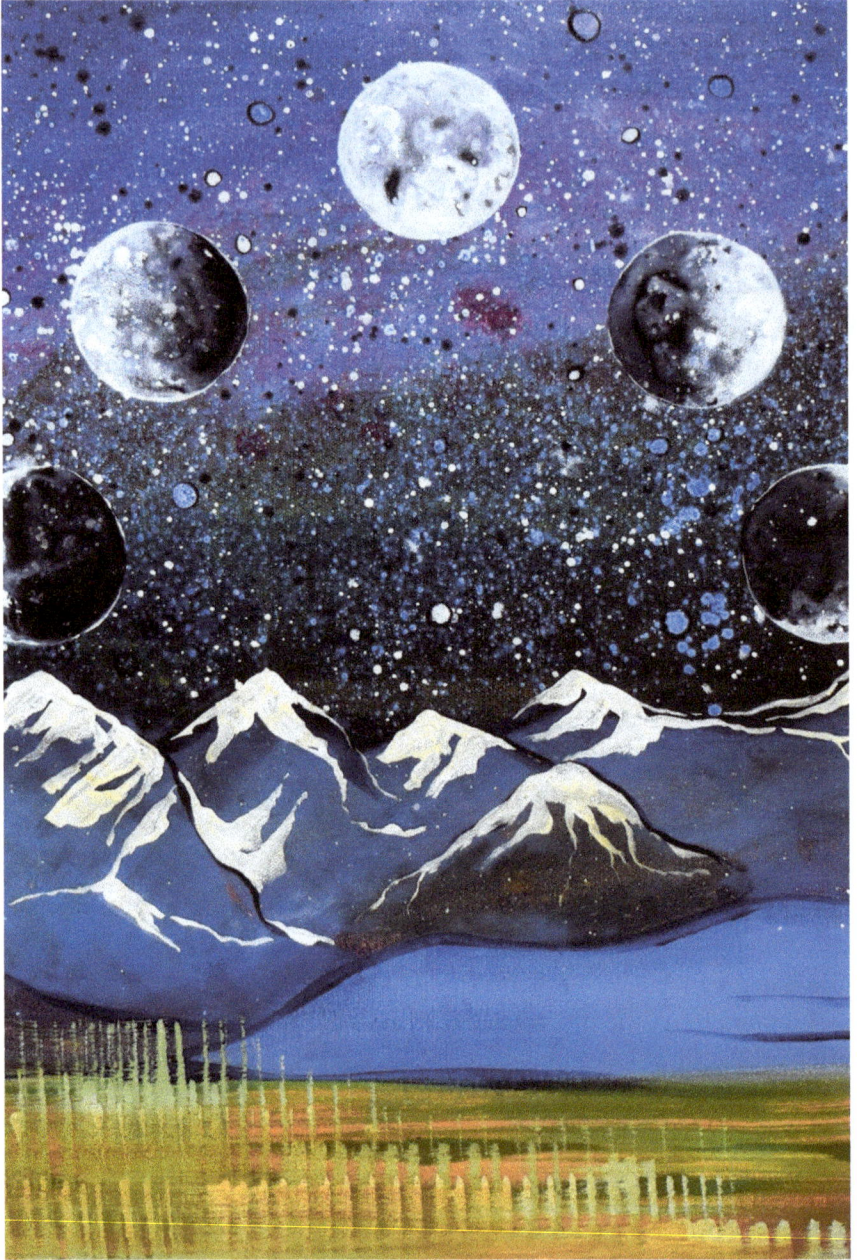

## Tend the Altar

In my part of the world, there is a damp and lasting darkness that happens during the final throes of November. Yes the days are growing shorter, but it's more than that. All autumn color has seeped away, revealing the charred brown and black of earth and the bruised gray and sepia of sky. The clouds roll in for weeks at a time and the mud and mess of early winter covers tires and boots and dogs and floorboards.

Then one day in early or mid-December as sunlight circles the drain of the year, the sky opens up and delivers light in the form of snow. What was once a blanket of dank decaying leaves transforms in an instant. Fresh fallen snow is a wonder to behold, not merely for its shocking whiteness, but for the light it reflects. The little bowl of our valley sheds its cave-like personality and becomes a mirror for the heavens.

## Altar Practice

I love winter in Pine Valley because it forces me to slow down and deeply notice the world around me. The cold compels you to contemplate, to deeply consider what you actually have energy for. There are no easy moments in winter. The fire burns only because you thought ahead, sawed the wood into rounds just the right size for your fire box, split it, hauled it, and sheltered it from the elements so that it would stay dry. The car starts only because you coddled it, let it warm up for a while, and shoveled a path out of the snowy bank that drifted in overnight. You have food on the table only because you planned ahead, drove an hour to the nearest town for groceries or grew it yourself in the heat of the summer months. So it's not easy. You must decide where you want to dedicate your energy.

And yet, there is ease. I never expected the pace of winter to be so wonderful. So silent. So comforting. So meditative. So joyful. Winter compresses the flow of daily life and brings you face to face with yourself. Winter asks that you remember who you are when the "busy" stops and the "have tos" fade. Winter says "stop and look around. Take time and keep your weight over your steady feet, else you slip on the ice."

All of the seeds produced during the last harvest are safely tucked beneath winter's protective snow cover. All but the pine cone. The pine cone endures the freezing temps of winter in exchange for exposure to sunlight, which is growing now day by day.

The pine cone's sacred geometry was recognized and revered by ancient cultures. The Mexican god "Chicomecoatl" is sometimes depicted with an offering of pine cones in one hand, and an evergreen tree in the other. Hindu deities are also often depicted holding a pine cone in an outstretched hand. The Egyptian Staff of Osiris (1224 BC) depicts two spiraling snakes rising up to meet at a pine cone. And Ancient Assyrian palace carvings (713-716 BC) depict winged people holding pine cones. All of these depictions seem to use the pine cone as a symbol of spiritual consciousness and enlightenment, awakening, or immortality.

For my ancestors the Celts, pine cones represented regeneration and were used as a fertility charm. They would place them under their pillows at night. And the ancient Romans associated pine cones with the goddess of love, Venus.

Speaking of Rome, the Catholic church uses the pine cone in its iconography as well. There is a pine cone carved into the holy staff that the Pope carries during religious ceremonies. And I'll never forget seeing the gargantuan bronze pine cone statue during a high school trip to the Vatican in Rome.

The pine cone itself is a marvel of creative momentum. An evolutionary precursor to the flower, pine cones fan out in a Fibonacci spiral sequence in either direction. Now, I'm not a math-person, but my high school geometry teacher, Mr. Schimke, explained to me that the Golden Spiral is a logarithmic spiral and its distinctiveness lies in the fact that it has Phi (golden ratio) as its growth factor. So for each quarter turn the spiral makes, it gets wider or away from the origin by a factor of Phi. Did you follow that? I can't quite connect to the math, but I can definitely connect to the visual.

The Golden Spiral and Golden Ratio are found everywhere in

nature, from the growth pattern of leaves and flowers to the sweeping curl of a nautilus to the spirals of galaxies. It's also how I experience creativity. Creativity has its own growth factor in that the more I engage my practice, the wider and more expansive it becomes. It sometimes takes great energy and faith to make that first move, but once you start, the exponential energy of creative practice can't help but spiral out from its center.

My altar for the winter solstice is full of pine cones in honor of their magic and symbolism. I hope that you too have a place to ritualize the magic of this amazing object and welcome the season of spiraling expansion, expanding creativity, and light.

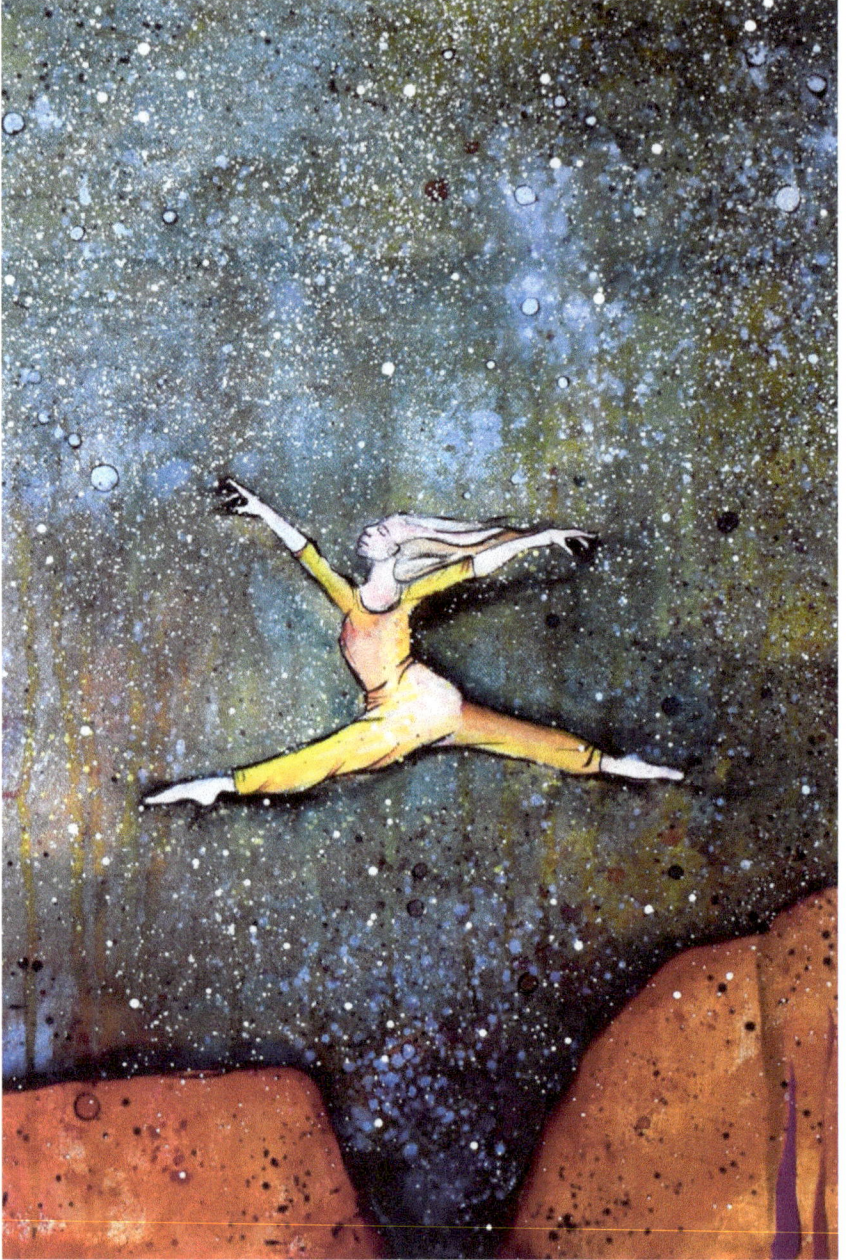

## Joy Practice

Samhain and Yule are seasonal twins. They complete each other. You can't truly understand one without the other. Just as Samhain explored the external shadows of the season and internal shadows of the soul, Yule highlights the outward illumination of the season and inner illumination of the spirit. I like thinking of Samhain as soul-work and Yule as spirit-work. Martin Shaw writes, "Spirit lifts. Soul deepens. Spirit is a spark; soul is a drop of water. Spirit is a great idea; soul is deep knowing. We absolutely need both."

## Incubation

**Where does SPIRIT show up in your life? What does it look, sound, smell, taste, feel like? As you write, let's actively recall our embodiment work from Beltane. Keep your observations grounded in the physical, sensual, tangible.**

**And same again for the soul. Where does SOUL show up in your life? What does it look, sound, smell, taste, and feel like? As you write, keep your observations grounded in the physical, sensual, tangible.**

If you haven't figured it out by now, I'm a witchy kind of person. My Irish and Scottish lineage, my nature-worshiping ways, and my goddess-centered outlook make for a potent Celtic cocktail of magic. This is how I think about my own soul and spirit work. In Gaelic, we refer to it as *Draíocht*. Draíocht (*pronounced DREE-oct*) literally means magic or enchantment. It sometimes denotes the secret lore and arts of the druids of pre-Christian Ireland and Celtic society. Much of my own joy and curiosity is rooted in the magic I find in Celtic myths and stories.

**Does your lineage have a magical strain or a mystical tradition? I bet it does! Do you feel drawn to that part of your lineage? Do you make**

room for ancestral wisdom and magic to move through you? How do you invite that kind of enchantment and healing into your life? Ritual? Art? Storytelling? Spell-casting? Chanting? Meditation?

## ACTION

I love reading the journals of other writers. It serves as a kind of creative conversation across time and space. The poet, essayist, and civil rights champion Audre Lorde published a series of diary entries in her book, *A Burst of Light: and Other Essays*, in which she stunningly addresses the purpose of her life. Her spirit shines through as she writes, "I want to live the rest of my life, however long or short, with as much sweetness as I can decently manage, loving all the people I love, and doing as much as I can of the work I still have to do. I am going to write fire until it comes out my ears, my eyes, my noseholes – everywhere. Until it's every breath I breathe. I'm going to go out like a fucking meteor!"

Let's grab our journals and write fire. This is no time to be shy. Audre Lorde had been diagnosed with terminal cancer when she wrote these words. We never know when our time will come, but this prompt is encouragement to get clear about how we'll spend the time we have "however long or short" that turns out to be.

**Writing fire was Audre Lorde's superpower. Where does your power lie? And more importantly, how do you use it in service of what you believe?**

As we write and sketch and sing and weave our work forward into Yule season, let's make sure that we are centering our own voice, spirit, and astonishment. In her book, *The Writing Life*, Annie Dillard says, "There is something you find interesting, for a reason hard to explain. It is hard to explain because you have never read it on any page; there you begin. You were made and set here to give voice to this, your own astonishment."

For me, it was the series of emotions I felt when a midwife transferred my newborn son from our home to the neonatal intensive care unit. After learning that my son was compromised and experiencing brain damage, I was stabilized by my midwife's assistant and then left alone in my own bedroom to make sense of my situation while the medical team followed my son to the hospital. I've never read or seen anything that resembles my astonishment surrounding that particular experience of solitude and personal reckoning. And I've always been curious about the ways in which I might tell that story.

**When have you been astonished by your own lived experience? Make a list.**

**Which parts of your inner world have you never read or seen? Is there an experience or thought process you've always longed to see reflected back to you? Make a list.**

**Your list may be short or long. It's no matter. Pick one and begin free-writing. Here are some opening lines that might help you get started:**

- **I can no longer conceal my astonishment about…**
- **Some things just have to be shared, which is why…**
- **I'm finally ready to reveal the truth of my experience of …**
- **Before I leave this earth, I have to tell you…**

~

The world is not a conglomeration of dead and inanimate objects. It is a thriving interconnected ecosystem. When we begin to make this critical shift in thinking we begin to see the truth and potency of the living web of relationships. This is the core insight of Earth-based spirituality. It is also what indigenous cultures have always maintained.

When we combine our deep understanding of interconnectedness with a creative practice that centers this web of relationship in all our choice-making, we arrive at a state I call Joy Mind. When we do this, our capacity for holding multiple truths increases. Joy Mind is a way to traverse liminal space and exist at our learning edge. I envision Joy

Mind as the Golden Spiral of the pinecone, doubling and re-doubling its capacity as it spirals out from its center. Joy Mind invites creative risk and resilience. When I actively cultivate Joy Mind, my creative work takes on a kind of mission-driven energy that endows my work with purpose, catalytic power, and capacity for connection. And when we awaken to the sacred interconnected web of all creation, and allow it to inform our creativity and choice-making, we can shift culture. The ancient Celts were acutely aware of this and their spiritual practices reflected this value.

What do I mean by *sacred*? Sacred does not mean something to which we worship or pay homage. The Sacred is what we value and acknowledge as essential and important. "Sacred" and "sacrifice" have the same root.

**What are you willing to risk or give up on your path towards greater right-relationship with the living earth?**

**And what are you committed to protecting or holding center on your path towards greater right-relationship with the living earth?**

## INTEGRATION

I wrote this book during the first blush of the Covid 19 pandemic. It was a time when we were unable to hug and hold each other. I longed for the connection of my family, my friends, and my community. So I developed a personal ritual informed by the Gaelic word, *Caim*. Caim means sanctuary, a prayer, or a circle casting. It is an invisible ring of protection, drawn around the body with the hand, to remind one of being safe and loved. So I used this Celtic idea of Caim (rhymes with lime) to practice a kind of socially distanced circle casting as a means of keeping us connected. Casting a circle is a form of prayer for protection, safety, and love. It is an easy way to create a sense of community even across time and distance.

The practice goes like this: Hold your distant loved one in your mind's eye or find them on an actual map. Envision a circle of light around both of your bodies. Envision a line of white light drawn on the earth that hurdles mountains and lakes and prairies and all manner of topography. It speeds towards your loved one, circles their body in space, and then circles back to you. The circle is cast. Breathe into the boundaries of that circle and fill it with warm light. Sense the expansiveness of your joy, of your light, and of your love. Let it radiate within the circle and on the body of your beloved. Speak their name and call them home to your heart. This is a powerful way of "holding" each other energetically, even when you cannot be in person and breathe the free air between you.

While you can practice Caim at any time, it is especially potent when combined with the solar return at this time of year. Model the action of the sun which shines longer and longer each day across larger and larger swaths of land. You are light energy. You are the Golden Spiral.

### ONE-WORD PROMPTS FOR YULE

Rebirth • Illuminate • Open • Pinecone • Source
Joy • Third Eye • Midnight • Candle • Gift
Glow • Truth • Poet • Sacred • Praise
Astonish • Solitude • Bell • Chorus • Reflect
Shine • Regeneration • Evergreen • Spiral • Cheer
Faith • Slow • Altar • Spirit • Child

### THE NEXT SIX WEEKS

The Gregorian calendar is coming to its end. A shiny new year is just around the corner. Over the next six weeks, rest. Resist the urge to make a list of resolutions. No need to jump up and "get going." It's still deep winter: a time of quiet contemplation, rather than one of active emergence. Notice the growing light. Reflect on the past year. Trust this sacred time of creative incubation.

### CROSS THE THRESHOLD

We are the roots, the water, the flowers, the fire, the sky, the seeds, the shadows, and all the light we can and cannot see. Not just us and them. We are them. They are us. This sacred interbeing is the gift of living on the ever-spinning Earth. This season, as the light breaks over winter's stark horizon, let's welcome the light with open arms and a heart full of hope.

Our creative work matters.
It is the thread with which we
intentionally mend the tattered bits
of this brokenhearted world.
Stitch by stitch by stitch.

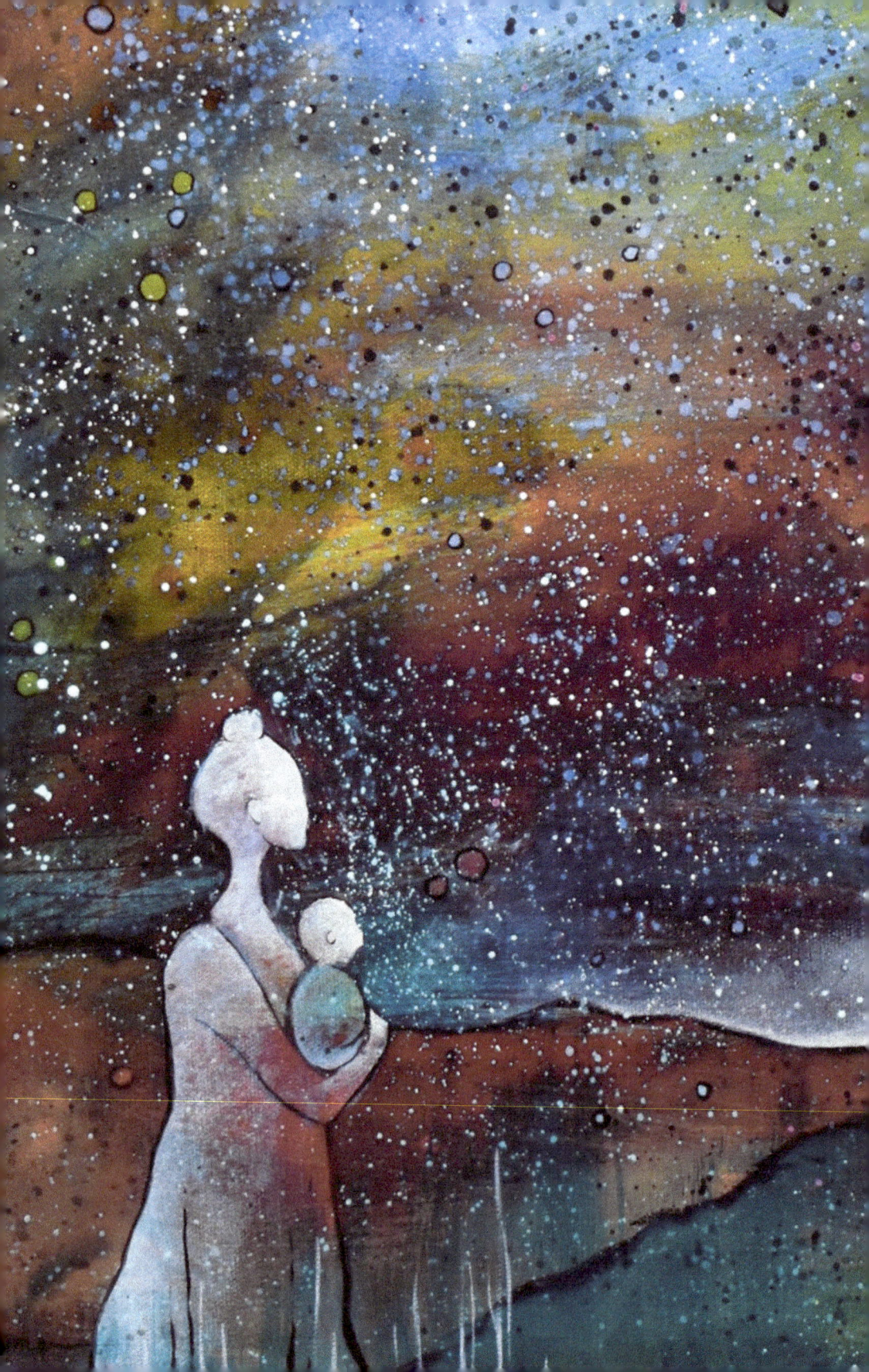

# 10

# CREATIVE ALCHEMY IN THE WILD

## Build Beloved Community

Have you ever witnessed a murmuration of starlings? It is a stunning thing to behold. I once saw one while visiting Town Lake in Austin, Texas. At first the birds looked like a soft, spinning tornado. The dark grouping then dropped, all at once, fanning out into a wide, undulating, intelligent cloud, pulsating just above the water. In an instant the birds, thousands of them, funneled together, and helix-like, carved the air into a vertical tube. Then, like school children released from class, the Starling cluster scattered from the top of the cylinder, only to gather again, forming an impossible feat of interlocking circles, swirling and plummeting towards Earth. I stood, gape-mouthed, and watched as they merged and separated, making silent music with their ever-evolving display of mutual movement. How did they do it? How do they do it without crashing into each other?

In 2010, Andrea Cavagna and the folks at the National Council of Research and the University of Rome used advanced computational modeling and video analysis to study how Starlings adjust to their flock mates. They determined that Starlings in large flocks consistently coordinate their movements with their seven nearest neighbors.

When one Starling changes direction or speed, each of the other birds in the flock responds to the change, and they do so nearly simultaneously regardless of the size of the flock. In essence, information moves across the flock very quickly and with nearly no degradation. The researchers describe it as a high signal-to-noise ratio. Signal-to-noise ratio can most simply be defined as more useful information (the signal) than unwanted data (the noise).

In her book *Emergent Strategy* (a seminal text for me about community organizing and social justice), adrienne maree brown writes about the Starling murmuration as a model for leaderless organization and collective action. But before we are able to create united murmurations in service of justice, we need self-aware birds that can communicate clear signals and trust what they see, hear, and feel. My highest hope for *The Creative Alchemy Cycle*, is not only that it helps us develop this level of clarity, trust, and awareness, but that we can merge our creative gifts and act in unison.

Building beloved community may seem like an overwhelming task, but just like our Starling sisters, we only need six or seven people around us to begin moving as one. As we greet the time before us, let's give ourselves permission to keep our circles small and focused. Let's practice loving kindness, deep trust, compassionate action, and right-relationship with those closest to us. Our liberation is bound together. It is interconnected, interdependent, and collective. As Starlings affect wide reaching change by tuning into their closest bird neighbors, so shall we make sweeping intentional change for the better. Empires fall. Institutions crumble. Corporations dissolve. But community? Community is ever-present.

We are at the beginning of what Joanna Macy calls a "great turning" — a cellular shift that summons human-kind to love one another back to wholeness. This call for healing comes not from some ethereal place, but directly from the Earth herself. And this is the essential adventure of our time: the shift from consumerist individualism to life-sustaining community practices.

The ills we face, the problems we must solve, the inequities we need to address - they all seem so overwhelming when consumed at once. Luckily, we can start where we are, as we are, and with only the resources currently available to us. And the best part is that we are not alone. There are scores of us, all across the globe, using our creative gifts to tell a new kind of story about our future. The answers to our most pressing questions do not lie in the hands of a single person. But when we live our truth in community, responding collectively, we become the answer we seek. We are Starlings for change. Our creative work in the world is the signal-to-noise ratio. Together, we are the murmuration.

### Set Your Work Free

I am a writer. I write every day. But the part that really trips me up about this life-long compulsion of mine, is that I am afraid to let you read it. I know this sounds counterintuitive because you're holding my book in your hands. But believe me when I tell you that this book is a monumental act of personal courage for me. I'm afraid that the inner workings of my heart and the thoughts that make up my beingness don't really matter or have no place in the wider discourse.

I feel the fear and do it anyway.

I share it because sharing completes the loop. Just as the brain sends out a signal for the hand to move — if the hand does not move, then the task is not complete and the brain fires off the message again. Sharing my writing is like the hand that follows the thought and completes the action. This is the full transmission. Then, and only then, can the brain rest. I don't know if this fear will ever go away. All I know is that I refuse to let it silence me.

The only way I know to empower our creative work is to set it free. Sharing our work with others has the potential to galvanize communities and invite them into a deep collective healing experience. It also allows us to excavate buried stories and shift dominant cultural narratives. Telling our own stories and sharing our own imagery is how we send signals to our closest flock mates.

### Your Joyful Work in the Wild

All along *The Creative Alchemy Cycle* journey, we've planted seeds.

We have developed a journal and sketchbook practice. What has flourished? What spoke to you? What creative ideas took root and grew strong and tall? We have also explored ways to embody our creative work and catalyze our activism and accountability. We have sung songs of gratitude, honored our collective grief, and centered creative nourishment and joy as our guidestars. But joy — finding it, feeling it, shouting it, and sharing it — joy above all else, is how we align with our values and connect with our communities.

Joy is not a luxury. It is not extra. It is a source of health, a birthright, built into the very cells of our beingness. Joy has a propulsive energy, capable of dismantling oppressive systems and shattering isolation. Joy is also a profound and unifying form of resistance. The force and momentum of liberatory movements is directly linked to our capacity and willingness to experience joy. Those who would suppress and oppress you, know this. That's why they want to squelch our joy.

Let us live and create with such joy that our very existence is an antidote to greed, inequity, exhaustion, depletion, extraction, disconnection, confusion, rage, hoarding, hate and lack. This is our moment, friends. Let us gather and channel our luminosity and energy, share our joy in whatever way we can, and become an uncontrollable force for good and right-relationship.

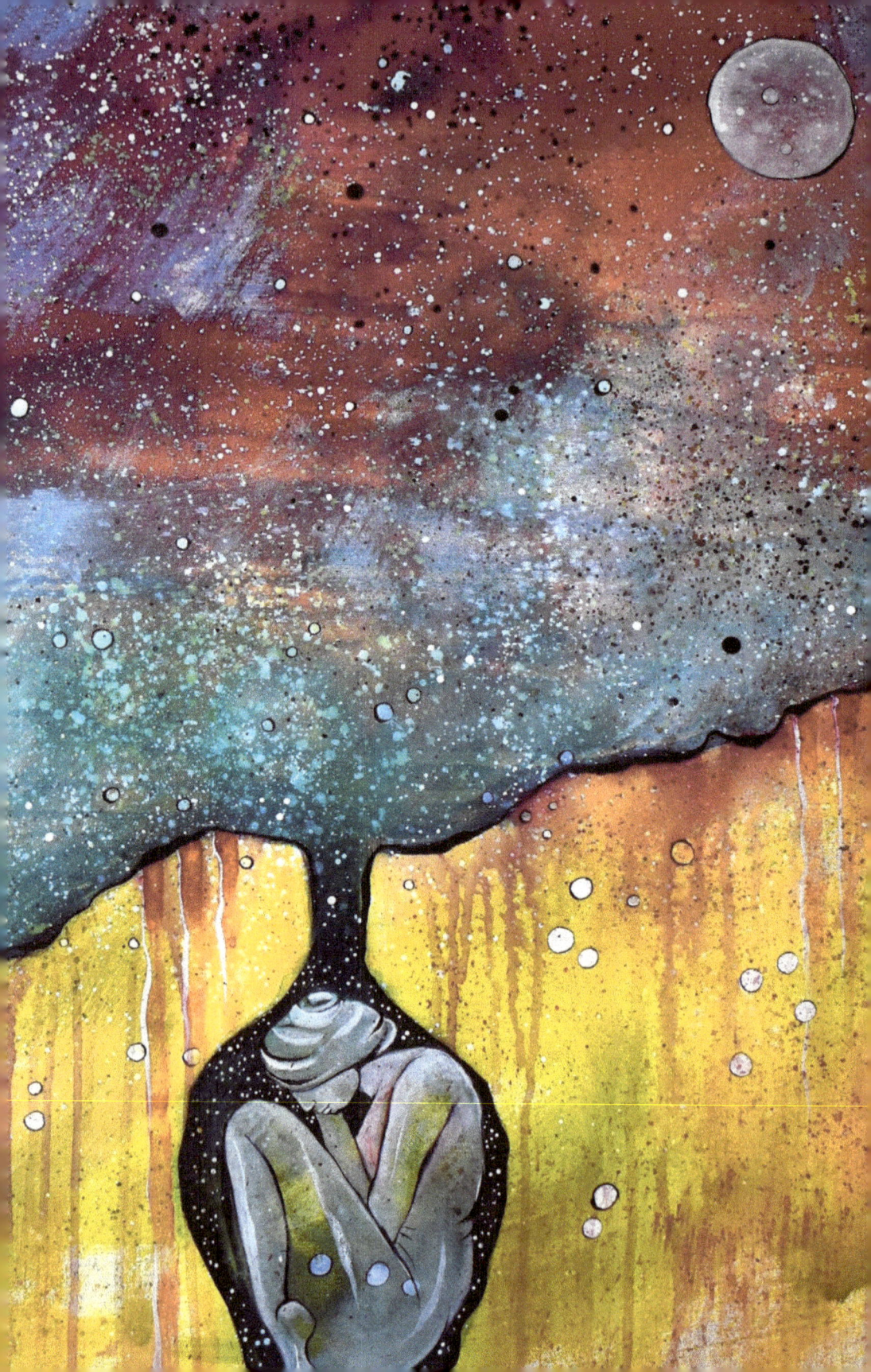

## 11

BEGIN AGAIN

Now that we've journeyed through *The Creative Alchemy Cycle* and experienced the potent energy of living in relationship to the Wheel of the Year, it's time to begin again.

This has been a catalytic year and I want to take a moment to honor all that you've accomplished. I also want to honor the rest and healing that has accompanied this work. The dial is moving. Change is at hand. We are a part of the centrifugal force of the great turning. We are joyfully powerful beyond our wildest imaginings. And we stand on the shoulders of giants – the ancestors who dreamed us into being. For them, we honor this moment. And I honor you. Here you are enough. Here you are held. Here you are whole.

Your innate creativity will transform the world.
Step into the center of your knowing
and alchemize your pain into joy.
It will set us all free.

# INDEX

We are a living expression of all we see, read, consume, and digest. As creatives, it is vital that we name the sources of our inspiration. These are the authors and texts that have influenced and shaped my creative process throughout *The Creative Alchemy Cycle*.

IMBOLC

- *The Art of Memoir* by Mary Karr
- *Bird by Bird: Some Instructions on Writing and Life* by Annie Lammott
- *Consolations: The Solace, Nourishment and Underlying Meaning of Everyday Words* by David Whyte
- *I Know Why the Caged Bird Sings* by Maya Angelou
- *Rest as Resistance: A Manifesto* by Tricia Hersey
- *The Writing Life* by Annie Dillard

OSTARA

- *Braiding Sweetgrass* by Robin Wall Kimmerer
- *Crazy Brave* by Joy Harjo

LUGHNASA

- *Conflict Resolution for Holy Beings: Poems* by Joy Harjo
- *Dreaming Accountability* by Mia Mingus
- *How to Be an Anti-Racist* by Ibram X. Kendi
- *The Sum of Us: What Racism Costs Everyone and How We Can Prosper Together* by Heather McGhee

MABON

- *Atlas of the Heart: Mapping Meaningful Connection and the Language of Human Experience* by Brené Brown
- *How To Eat* by Thich Nhat Hanh
- *Women Who Run With the Wolves: Myths and Stories of the Wild Woman Archetype* by Clarissa Pinkola Estés

SAMHAIN

- *Active Hope (revised): How to Face the Mess We're in with Unexpected Resilience and Creative Power* by Joanna Macy & Chris Johnstone
- *Courting the Wild Twin* by Martin Shaw
- *What it Takes to Heal: How Transforming Ourselves Can Change the World* by Prentis Hemphill
- *When Things Fall Apart: Heart Advice for Difficult Times* by Pema Chödrön
- *Prayers of Honoring Voice* by Pixie Lighthorse

YULE

- *Bless The Space Between Us* by John O'Donohue
- *Letters to a Young Poet* by Rainer Maria Rilke
- *A Responsibility to Awe* by Rebeca Elson
- *Wintering: The Power of Rest and Retreat in Difficult Times* by Katherine May

# IMAGE KEY

All original artwork by Sarah Greenman

# A NOTE ON STORIES

I am a listener and have been collecting stories and anecdotes as long as I've had a journal. Stories shared in this book that are not my own were shared with permission, and some names have been changed. I share these stories here with awe, respect, love and gratitude.

# ACKNOWLEDGMENTS

A deep bow of gratitude for the Eastern Oregon landscape that birthed this book. For the Wallowa Whitman mountain range that sheltered my dreaming. For my daily writing companion, the Douglas fir at the far edge of my front yard. For the orchard along Eagle Creek that held me and nourished me, the Canyon Wren who reminded me to use my voice, and the high desert sage that invited me again and again to pause, listen, and learn.

Thank you to Anya Hankin for your incredible mentorship and for fanning the flames of this work when it was a tiny spark. Thank you to Myriam Loeschen for your wise and generous words of encouragement and enduring friendship. Thank you to Heather Dakota for stepping in as the first editor to work with this volume of disparate stories, always bringing me back to the core question at hand.

To my parents Connie Atkinson and John Lambie and my grandmothers Jane Lambie and Orma Minshull, whose love, artistry, and unending faith in my creativity is the foundation upon which I lay the building blocks of my life. There are not thanks enough for the support they have given me.

To Jack Greenman, the father of my children and my creative partner for 20 years. Our marriage may not have been one for the ages, but our creative collaborations are. Thank you for nurturing this book and for your incredible good company and tender care.

This book emerged during a series of writing cohorts and workshops and would not be in the hands of readers today without the phenomenal insight and collaboration of Rowen White, Caitlin Quinn, B Merikle, Jenny Downer, kacy borba spann, Clare Kritter, Marisol Cordero Goodman, and Amy McMullen.

The pages of this book bloomed during the first years of a global pandemic when a group of intrepid, heart-centered creatives joined me for a year-long journey. To the 150-plus fellow travelers who interacted online with *The Creative Alchemy Cycle* from 2020-2024, you have my deep gratitude. Thank you for walking this path alongside me.

To Kelly Madding, thank you for your unconditional love, your unwavering belief in my work, and for running the last leg of this journey with me.

Special thanks to Angela Yarber for believing in my book and guiding this manuscript to publication.

# ABOUT THE AUTHOR

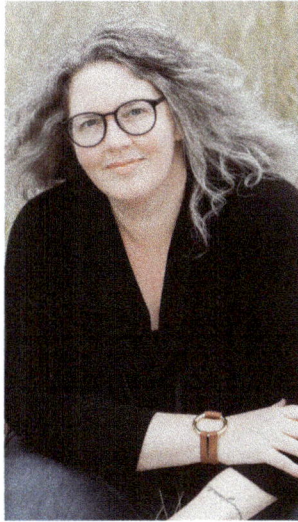

SARAH GREENMAN is an artist, story-teller, theater-maker, facilitator, mother, and community organizer. Her work has appeared in a range of publications, including *The Huffington Post*, *Advocate*, *Texas Monthly*, *D Magazine*, *Curbed*, *Elle Décor*, *Spirituality & Health*, *Houzz*, *Apartment Therapy*, and *Country Decorating*. Her plays have been produced in New York, Seattle, Dallas, Berkely, and Oakland. She lives in rural Oregon.

www.sarahgreenman.com